HANDBOOK of COMMONLY PRESCRIBED PEDIATRIC DRUGS

Sixth Edition

Edward J. Barbieri, Ph.D.
National Medical Services
Willow Grove, Pennsylvania
and
Adjunct Associate Professor of Pharmacology
MCP Hahnemann University
Philadelphia, Pennsylvania

Felicia Corsaro-Barbieri, Ph.D.
Professor of Chemistry
School of Arts and Sciences
Gwynedd-Mercy College
Gwynedd Valley, Pennsylvania

G. John DiGregorio, M.D., Ph.D.
National Medical Services
Willow Grove, Pennsylvania
and
Professor of Pharmacology and Medicine
MCP Hahnemann University
Philadelphia, Pennsylvania

1999

HANDBOOK OF COMMONLY PRESCRIBED PEDIATRIC DRUGS

Sixth Edition

The **HANDBOOK OF COMMONLY PRESCRIBED PEDIATRIC DRUGS, Sixth Edition,** *attempts to present the most common trade names and pediatric doses, and should be used only as a guideline to these; it should not be considered as an official therapeutic document. If there is a discrepancy in therapeutic category, preparations, and dosages, the reader is advised to obtain official and more complete information from the pharmaceutical manufacturer.*

The Authors or Publisher are not responsible for typographical errors within the contents of this booklet.

PREFACE

We are pleased to present the **Sixth Edition** of the **HANDBOOK OF COMMONLY PRESCRIBED PEDIATRIC DRUGS**. It has been almost four years since the last edition was published, and a significant number of changes were made to improve the present edition. All tables have been revised with the latest available information on drugs and drug products; we estimate that over 100 new therapeutic agents have been added. Many products with new therapeutic indications for children as well as many new dosage formulations have been included. Moreover, a few new therapeutic categories of drugs, e.g., Antacids, Drugs for Cystitis Fibrosis, Drugs for Obsessive-Compulsive Disorder, and Keratolytics, have been added.

The tables on Immune Serums, Bacterial Vaccines, and Viral Vaccines have all been extensively revised and expanded. The Nutritional Section has been completely revised to, hopefully, a more useful form.

As always, we have prepared the **HANDBOOK OF COMMONLY PRESCRIBED PEDIATRIC DRUGS, Sixth Edition** in an attempt to present the most common trade names and pediatric dosages. However, the use of drugs in therapy is constantly being modified due to acquired knowledge obtained through new research data, clinical experiences, and approaches to the treatment of diseases in patients. In addition, the drug preparations that are available are continually changing. We have checked sources believed to be reliable for the purpose of providing information that is appropriate and that reflects the general standards of practice accepted at the time of this publication. Nevertheless, the drug preparations and the dosages contained in this handbook should be used only as guidelines and the text should not to be considered as an official therapeutic document. If there is a discrepancy in preaparation or dosage, the reader is advised to obtain official and more complete information from the pharmaceutical manufacturer.

We sincerely hope that this handbook becomes a valuable companion that will enhance your familiarity with drugs and drug prescribing for children. Please feel free to contact us with any suggestions, comments, and criticisms that you might have.

Edward J. Barbieri, Ph.D.
Felicia Corsaro-Barbieri, Ph.D.
G. John DiGregorio, M.D., Ph.D.

TABLE OF CONTENTS

THERAPEUTIC CATEGORY LISTING[a]

[a] This section lists, by Therapeutic Category, drugs found in the **SELECTED INDIVIDUAL DRUG PREPARATIONS** (pp. 19 to 109) and the **SELECTED COMBINATION DRUG PREPARATIONS** (pp. 111 to 152) sections only. Refer to the **INDEX** for a more complete listing of drugs.

Drug names in UPPER CASE represent TRADE NAMES; the TRADE NAMES without generic names preceeding them are COMBINATION PRODUCTS.

1

2

3

4

9

16

Notes

SELECTED

INDIVIDUAL

DRUG

PREPARATIONS

GENERIC NAME	COMMON TRADE NAMES	THERAPEUTIC CATEGORY	PREPARATIONS	COMMON PEDIATRIC DOSAGE
Acetaminophen	INFANTS' TYLENOL	Non-Opioid Analgesic, Antipyretic	Solution (Drops): 80 mg/0.8 mL	0-3 mos (6-11 lbs): 0.4 mL q 4 h po. 4-11 mos (12-17 lbs): 0.8 mL q 4 h po. 1-2 yrs (18-23 lbs): 1.2 mL q 4 h po. 2-3 yrs (24-35 lbs): 1.6 mL q 4 h po. For all of the above, do not exceed 5 doses within 24 h.
	CHILDREN'S TYLENOL		Susp. & Elixir: 160 mg/5 mL	4-11 mos (12-17 lbs): 2.5 mL q 4 h po. 12-23 mos (18-23 lbs): 3.75 mL q 4 h po.
			Chewable Tab: 80 mg	2-3 yrs (24-35 lbs): 2 tabs or 5 mL q 4 h po. 4-5 yrs (36-47 lbs): 3 tabs or 7.5 mL q 4 h po. 6-8 yrs (48-59 lbs): 4 tabs or 10 mL q 4 h po. 9-10 yrs (60-71 lbs): 5 tabs or 12.5 mL q 4 h po. 11 yrs (72-95 lbs): 6 tabs or 15 mL q 4 h po. For all of the above, do not exceed 5 doses within 24 h.
	TEMPRA QUICKLETS (Children's Strength)		Chewable Tabs: 80 mg	Same doses as for CHILDREN'S TYLENOL Chewable Tablets above.
	JUNIOR STRENGTH TYLENOL		Cplt & Chewable Tab: 160 mg	6-8 yrs (48-59 lbs): 2 cplts or tabs q 4 h po. 9-10 yrs (60-71 lbs): 2.5 cplts or tabs q 4 h po. 11 yrs (72-95 lbs): 3 cplts or tabs q 4 h po. 12 yrs (over 95 lbs): 4 cplts or tabs q 4 h po. For all of the above, do not exceed 5 doses within 24 h.
	TEMPRA QUICKLETS (Junior Strength)		Chewable Tabs: 160 mg	Same doses as for TYLENOL JUNIOR STRENGTH Chewable Tablets above.
	TYLENOL (Regular (Strength)		Cplt & Tab: 325 mg	6-11 yrs: 1/2 - 1 cplt or tab q 4 - 6 h po. not to exceed 5 doses in 24 h. 12 yrs: 2 cplts or tabs q 4 - 6 h po, not to exceed 5 doses in 24 h.

	INFANT'S FEVERALL	**Rectal Suppos**: 80 mg	**3-11 mos**: Insert 1 rectally q 6 h. **1-3 yrs**: Insert 1 rectally q 4 h.
	CHILDREN'S FEVERALL	**Rectal Suppos**: 120 mg	**3-6 yrs**: Insert 1 rectally q 4 - 6 h.
	JUNIOR STRENGTH FEVERALL	**Rectal Suppos**: 325 mg	**6-12 yrs**: Insert 1 rectally q 4 - 6 h.
Acetic Acid	DOMEBORO	Antibacterial, Antifungal	**Otic Solution**: 2%	Patient should lie on his side with affected ear uppermost. Instill 4 - 6 drops into the ear canal and maintain this position for 5 min. Repeat the process q 2 - 3 h.
	VOSOL		**Otic Solution**: 2%	Carefully remove all cerumen and debris. Insert a wick saturated with the solution into the ear canal. Keep in for at least 24 h and keep moist by adding 3 - 5 drops of solution q 4 - 6 h.
Acetylcysteine Sodium	MUCOMYST, MUCOSIL	Mucolytic	**Solution**: 10, 20%	**Nebulization (tracheostomy, mask or mouth** **piece)**: 3 - 5 mL (of 20% solution) or 6 - 10 mL (of 10% solution) tid to qid. **Direct Instillation**: 1 - 2 mL (of 10 or 20% solution) as often as every hour.
Acyclovir	ZOVIRAX	Antiviral	**Cpsl**: 200 mg **Susp**: 200 mg/5 mL **Tab**: 400, 800 mg	**Chickenpox (Over 2 yrs and < 40 kg)**: 20 mg/kg (not to exceed 800 mg) qid po for 5 days. **Chickenpox (Over 2 yrs and > 40 kg)**: 800 mg qid po for 5 days.

GENERIC NAME	COMMON TRADE NAMES	THERAPEUTIC CATEGORY	PREPARATIONS	COMMON PEDIATRIC DOSAGE
Acyclovir Sodium	ZOVIRAX	Antiviral	**Powd for Inj:** 500, 1000 mg	**Mucosal and Cutaneous Herpes simplex Infections in Immunocompromised Patients (Under 12 yrs):** 250 mg/m^2 infused IV at a constant rate over 1 h, q 8 h for 7 days. **Herpes simplex Encephalitis (6 mos - 12 yrs):** 500 mg/m^2 infused IV at a constant rate over at least 1 h, q 8 h for 10 days. **Varicella zoster in Immunocompromised Patients (Under 12 yrs):** 500 mg/m^2 infused IV at a constant rate over at least 1 h, q 8 h for 7 days.
Albendazole	ALBENZA	Anthelmintic	**Tab:** 200 mg	**Hydatid Disease:** Administer in a 28-day cycle followed by a 14-day albendazole-free interval, for a total of 3 cycles. < 60 kg: 15 mg/kg/day po in divided doses (bid) with meals (maximum: 800 mg/day). ≥ 60 kg: 400 mg bid po with meals. **Neurocysticercosis:** Administer for 8 - 30 days. < 60 kg: 15 mg/kg/day po in divided doses (bid) with meals (maximum: 800 mg/day). ≥ 60 kg: 400 mg bid po with meals.
Albuterol	VENTOLIN	Bronchodilator	**Aerosol:** 90 μg/spray	**Over 4 yrs:** 1 - 2 inhalations repeated q 4 - 6 h.
Albuterol Sulfate	VENTOLIN, PROVENTIL	Bronchodilator	**Syrup:** 2 mg (of albuterol base)/5 mL	**2-6 yrs:** Usually 0.1 mg/kg tid po. Maximum: 2 mg tid. For those who do not respond satisfactorily, the dose may be increased stepwise to 0.2 mg/kg tid, but not to exceed 4 mg tid. **6-14 yrs:** Usually 2 mg tid or qid po. For those who do not respond to 2 mg qid, the dose may be cautiously increased stepwise, but not to exceed 24 mg per day (given in divided doses).

	VENTOLIN		**Tab:** 2, 4 mg (of albuterol base)	**6-12 yrs:** Usually 2 mg tid or qid po. For those who do not respond favorably to 2 mg qid, the dose may be cautiously increased stepwise, but not to exceed 24 mg per day (given in divided doses).
			Inhalation Solution: 0.5% (as albuterol base)	**2-12 yrs:** Initially 0.1 - 0.15 mg/kg/dose, with subsequent dosing titrated to achieved the desired clinical response. Do not exceed 2.5 mg tid - qid by nebulization.
	VENTOLIN NEBULES		**Inhalation Solution:** 0.083% (as albuterol base) in in 3 mL nebules	**2-12 yrs (and at least 15 kg):** 1 nebule (2.5 mg) tid - qid by nebulization.
	VENTOLIN ROTACAPS		**Cpsl for Inhalation:** 200 μg	**Over 4 yrs:** Usually 200 μg inhaled q 4 - 6 h using a Rotahaler inhalation device. In some, 400 μg inhaled q 4 - 6 h may be required.
Alclometasone Dipropionate	ACLOVATE	Corticosteroid	**Cream & Oint:** 0.05%	**Over 1 yr:** Apply a thin film to affected skin areas bid to tid; massage in gently until the medication disappears.
Alprostadil	PROSTIN VR PEDIATRIC	Prostaglandin	**Inj:** 500 μg/mL	Initially 0.05 - 0.1 μg/kg/min by continuous IV infusion. Dose may be increased up to 0.4 μg/kg/min IV to achieve the desired effect, then reduce the infusion rate to provide the lowest possible dose that maintains the desired response.
Amantadine Hydrochloride	SYMMETREL	Antiviral	**Syrup:** 50 mg/5 mL **Cpsl:** 100 mg	**1-9 yrs:** 2 - 4 mg/lb/day (4.4 - 8.8 mg/kg/day) given once daily or bid po; not to exceed 150 mg/day. **Over 9 yrs:** 100 mg bid po.
Amcinonide	CYCLOCORT	Corticosteroid	**Cream & Oint:** 0.1% **Lotion:** 0.1%	Apply to affected areas bid to tid. Rub into affected areas bid.

GENERIC NAME	COMMON TRADE NAMES	THERAPEUTIC CATEGORY	PREPARATIONS	COMMON PEDIATRIC DOSAGE
Amikacin Sulfate	AMIKIN	Antibacterial	Inj (per mL): 50, 250 mg	**Newborns:** It is recommended that a loading dose of 10 mg/kg IM be administered initially, followed by 7.5 mg/kg q 12 h IM or by IV infusion (over 1 - 2 hours). **Older Neonates & Children:** 15 mg/kg/day in equally divided doses q 8 - 12 h IM or by IV infusion (over 30 - 60 minutes).
Aminophylline		Bronchodilator	Liquid: 105 mg/5 mL Tab: 100, 200 mg Inj: 250 mg/10 mL	See the Oral Aminophylline Table, p. 160. See the Oral Aminophylline Table, p. 160. See the IV Aminophylline Table, p. 161.

Amoxicillin	AMOXIL	Antibacterial	Powd for Susp (Drops): 50 mg/mL	**Infections of the Lower Respiratory Tract and**
				  Under 6 kg (13 lbs): 1.25 mL q 8 h po.
				  6-7 kg (13-15 lbs): 1.75 mL q 8 h po.
				  8 kg (16-18 lbs): 2.25 mL q 8 h po.
				All Other Infections and
				  Under 6 kg (13 lbs): 0.75 mL q 8 h po.
				  6-7 kg (13-15 lbs): 1.0 mL q 8 h po.
				  8 kg (16-18 lbs): 1.25 mL q 8 h po.

	AMOXIL, WYMOX		Powd for Susp (per 5 mL): 125, 250 mg
			Cpsl: 250, 500 mg
				Infections of the Lower Respiratory Tract and
				  Under 20 kg: 40 mg/kg/day in divided doses q 8 h po.
				  Over 20 kg: 500 mg q 8 h po.

	AMOXIL		Chewable Tab: 125, 250 mg	**Infections of the Ear, Nose and Throat; Skin and Soft Tissues; or Genitourinary Tract and**
				  Under 20 kg: 20 - 40 mg/kg/day in divided doses q 8 h po.
				  Over 20 kg: 250 - 500 mg q 8 h po.
				Gonorrheal Infections, Acute Uncomplicated: Prepubertal Children: 50 mg/kg combined with 25 mg/kg probenecid po as a single dose.

Amphetamine Sulfate (C-II)		CNS Stimulant	**Tab:** 5 mg	**Attention Deficit Disorder:** **3-6 yrs:** Initially 2.5 mg per day po; the dose may be raised by 2.5 mg each week to a maximum of 60 mg per day. **Over 6 yrs:** Double the above dosage schedule. Maximum: 60 mg/day.
Amphotericin B	FUNGIZONE ORAL SUSPENSION	Antifungal	**Susp:** 100 mg/mL	1 mL qid po. If possible, administer between meals (for longer contact with the oral lesions).
	FUNGIZONE		**Cream, Lotion & Oint:** 3%	Apply topically bid - qid.
Amphotericin B Cholesteryl Sulfate Complex	AMPHOTEC	Antifungal	**Powd for Inj:** 50, 100 mg	Initially, 3 - 4 mg/kg/day by slow IV infusion (rate 1 mg/kg/h) diluted in 5% Dextrose for Injection. A test dose immediately before the first dose is advisable when beginning all new courses of treatment.
Amphotericin B Lipid Complex	ABELCET	Antifungal	**Powd for Inj:** 100 mg	5 mg/kg daily as a single IV infusion at a rate of 2.5 mg/kg/h.
Ampicillin Anhydrous	OMNIPEN	Antibacterial	**Powd for Susp (per 5 mL):** 125, 250 mg **Cpsl:** 250, 500 mg	**Respiratory Tract and Soft Tissue Infections:** **Under 20 kg:** 50 mg/kg/day in divided doses q 6 - 8 h po. **Over 20 kg:** 250 mg q 6 h po. **Genitourinary or Gastrointestinal Infections:** **Under 20 kg:** 100 mg/kg/day in divided doses q 6 h po. **Over 20 kg:** 500 mg q 6 h po.

GENERIC NAME	COMMON TRADE NAMES	THERAPEUTIC CATEGORY	PREPARATIONS	COMMON PEDIATRIC DOSAGE
Ampicillin Sodium	OMNIPEN-N	Antibacterial	Powd for Inj: 125, 250, 500 mg; 1, 2 g	**Neonates (Birth - 7 days):** 25 mg/kg/day in divided doses q 12 h IM or IV. **For Meningitis:** 50 mg/kg q 6 h IM or IV. **Neonates (Over 7 days):** 25 mg/kg/day in divided doses q 8 h IM or IV. **For Meningitis:** 50 mg/kg q 6 h IM or IV. **Respiratory Tract and Soft Tissue Infections: Under 40 kg:** 25 - 50 mg/kg/day in equally divided doses at 6 - 8 h intervals IM or IV. **Over 40 kg:** 250 - 500 mg q 6 h IM or IV. **Genitourinary or Gastrointestinal Tract Infections including Gonorrhea in Females: Under 40 kg:** 50 mg/kg/day in equally divided doses at 6 - 8 h intervals IM or IV. **Over 40 kg:** 500 mg q 6 h IM or IV. **Prevention of Bacterial Endocarditis (for Dental, or Upper Respiratory Tract Procedures): At Moderate Risk:** 50 mg/kg (up to 2 g) IM or IV, 30 min. prior to the procedure. **At High Risk:** 50 mg/kg (up to 2 g) IM or IV + gentamicin 1.5 mg/kg, 30 min. prior to the procedure. 6 h later: ampicillin 25 mg/kg IM or IV or 25 mg/kg po.
Ampicillin Trihydrate	PRINCIPEN	Antibacterial	Cpsl: 250, 500 mg Powd for Susp (per 5 mL): 125, 250 mg	Same po dosages as for OMNIPEN above.
Asparaginase	ELSPAR	Antineoplastic	Powd for Inj: 10,000 IUnits	200 IU/kg/day IV (over a 30 minute period) for 28 days.

Aspirin	BAYER CHILDREN'S ASPIRIN	Non-Opioid Analgesic, Antipyretic, Nonsteroidal Anti-Inflammatory Drug	**Chewable Tab:** 81 mg	**Analgesic and Antipyretic:** 65 mg/kg/day in 4 - 6 divided doses po or rectally. **Doses by age and weight:** **2-4 yrs (32-35 lbs):** 2 tabs q 4 h po. **4-6 yrs (36-45 lbs):** 3 tabs q 4 h po. **6-9 yrs (46-65 lbs):** 4 tabs q 4 h po. **9-11 yrs (66-76 lbs):** 4-5 tabs q 4 h po. **11-12 yrs (77-83 lbs):** 4-6 tabs q 4 h po. **12 yrs & Older:** 5-8 tabs q 4 h po. For all of the above, do not exceed 5 doses within 24 h. **Antirheumatic:** 100 mg/kg/day in 4 - 6 divided doses po.
			Tab & Cplt: 325 mg	Please see the Aspirin Table, p. 156.
			Rectal Suppos: 60 to 650 mg	Variable depending on the child's age and weight.
Atracurium Besylate	TRACRIUM INJECTION	Neuromuscular Blocker	**Inj:** 10 mg/mL	**1 mo - 2 yrs:** 0.3 - 0.4 mg/kg as an IV bolus is recommended as the initial dose under halothane anesthesia. **Over 2 yrs:** 0.4 - 0.5 mg/kg as an IV bolus when used alone; 0.25 - 0.35 mg/kg as an IV bolus when used under steady state with certain general anesthetics. Doses of 0.08 to 0.10 mg/kg for maintenance during prolonged surgery. Maintenance doses may be required with slightly greater frequency in infants and children than in adults.
Atropine Sulfate		Anticholinergic	**Soluble Tab:** 0.4, 0.6 mg **Inj (per mL):** 0.05 to 1.0 mg	**Antisialogogue in Surgery:** **Infants Under 5 kg:** 0.04 mg/kg q 4 - 6 h IV, IM or SC. **Infants Over 5 kg:** 0.03 mg/kg q 4 - 6 h IV, IM or SC. **Older Children:** 0.01 mg/kg q 4 - 6 h po, IV, IM or SC. Maximum: 0.4 mg/dose.

[Continued on the next page]

GENERIC NAME	COMMON TRADE NAMES	THERAPEUTIC CATEGORY	PREPARATIONS	COMMON PEDIATRIC DOSAGE
Atropine Sulfate [Continued]	ISOPTO ATROPINE	Mydriatic - Cycloplegic	Ophth Sol: 0.5, 1%	**Uveitis:** 1 - 2 drops of the 0.5% solution in the affected eye(s) up to tid. Compress inner canthus for 1 min to reduce absorption.
	ATROPINE SULFATE S.O.P.		Ophth Oint: 0.5, 1%	**Uveitis:** Apply to eye(s) up to bid.
Attapulgite	DONNAGEL	Antidiarrheal	Liquid: 600 mg/15 mL (1.4% alcohol) Chewable Tab: 600 mg	**3-5 yrs:** 7.5 mL or 1/2 tab po at the first sign of diarrhea, and repeat after each subsequent bowel movement. Maximum: 7 doses per 24 hours. **6-11 yrs:** double the above dose. Maximum: 7 doses per per hours.
	PAREPECTOLIN		Liquid: 600 mg/15 mL	**3-6 yrs:** 7.5 mL po after each bowel movement, up to 7 times daily. **6-12 yrs:** 15 mL po after each bowel movement, up to 7 times daily.
	KAOPECTATE		Liquid: 750 mg/15 mL Cplt: 750 mg	**3-6 yrs:** 7.5 mL po at the first sign of diarrhea and after each subsequent bowel movement. Maximum: 7 doses per 24 hours. **6-12 yrs:** 15 mL (or 1 cplt) po at the first sign of diarrhea and after each subsequent bowel movement. Maximum: 7 doses of Liquid or 6 cplts per 24 hours.
	DIASORB		Liquid: 750 mg/5 mL Tab: 750 mg	**3-6 yrs:** 5 mL or 1 tab po at the first sign of diarrhea, and repeat after each subsequent bowel movement. Maximum: 3 doses per 24 hours. **6-12 yrs:** double the above dose. Maximum: 3 doses per 24 hours.
	RHEABAN		Cplt: 750 mg	**6-12 yrs:** 1 cplt po after the initial bowel movement; 1 cplt after each subsequent bowel movement. Maximum: 6 cplts per 24 hours.

Aurothioglucose	SOLGANAL	Antiarthritic	Inj: 50 mg/mL	**6-12 yrs:** One-fourth of the adult dose, governed chiefly by body weight, not to exceed 25 mg per dose. **Adult dose:** First dose: 10 mg IM; second and third doses: 25 mg IM; fourth and subsequent doses: 50 mg IM. The interval between doses is 1 week. The 50 mg dose is continued at weekly intervals until 0.8 to 1.0 g has been given. If the patient has improved and shows no sign of toxicity, the 50 mg dose may be continued for many months longer, at 3 - 4 week intervals.
Azithromycin Dihydrate	ZITHROMAX	Antibacterial	Powd for Susp (per 5 mL): 100, 200 mg Cpsl: 250 mg	**Acute Otitis Media and Community-acquired Pneumonia (Over 6 mos):** 10 mg/kg as a single dose on the first day (not to exceed 500 mg) followed by 5 mg/kg (not to exceed 250 mg) on days 2 through 5. Administer on an empty stomach. **Pharyngitis/Tonsillitis (Over 2 yrs):** 12.5 mg/kg po as a single dose (not to exceed 500 mg) for 5 days. Administer on an empty stomach.
Aztreonam	AZACTAM	Antibacterial	Powd for Inj: 0.5, 1, 2 g	**Over 9 mos (Mild-to-Moderate Infections):** 30 mg/kg q 8 h by IV infusion. Maximum: 120 mg/kg/day. **Over 9 mos (Moderate-to-Severe Infections):** 30 mg/kg q 6 or 8 h by IV infusion. Maximum: 120 mg/kg/day.
Bacampicillin Hydrochloride	SPECTROBID	Antibacterial	Tab: 400 mg	**Upper Respiratory Tract Infections, Urinary Tract Infections, Skin and Skin Structure Infections (≥ 25 kg):** 25 mg/kg/day po in 2 equally divided doses at 12 h intervals. **Lower Respiratory Tract Infections and Severe Infections (≥ 25 kg):** 50 mg/kg/day po in 2 equally divided doses at 12 h intervals.

GENERIC NAME	COMMON TRADE NAMES	THERAPEUTIC CATEGORY	PREPARATIONS	COMMON PEDIATRIC DOSAGE
Bacitracin		Antibacterial	Ophth Oint: 500 Units/g	Apply to affected eye(s) 1 or more times daily.
			Oint: 500 Units/g	Apply topically to the affected areas 1 - 3 times daily.
Barley Malt Extract	MALTSUPEX	Bulk Laxative	Liquid: 16 grams/15 mL	**1 mo - 2 yrs:** 1 - 2 teaspoonfuls (5 - 10 mL) in water, fruit juice, or formula bid - tid po. **2-6 yrs:** 1/2 tablespoonful (7.5 mL) in 8 fl. oz. of liquid bid po. **6-12 yrs:** 1 tablespoonful (15 mL) in 8 fl. oz. of liquid bid po.
			Powder: 8 g/level scoop	**1 mo - 2 yrs:** 2 - 3 level teaspoonfuls in water, fruit juice, or formula tid - qid po. **2-6 yrs:** 1 scoop bid po. Drink a full glass (8 fl. oz.) of liquid with each dose. **6-12 yrs:** Up to 2 scoops bid po. Drink a full glass (8 fl. oz.) of liquid with each dose.
Beclomethasone Dipropionate	BECLOVENT, VANCERIL	Corticosteroid	Aerosol: 42 μg/spray	**6-12 yrs:** 1 - 2 inhalations tid or qid.
	VANCERIL DOUBLE STRENGTH		Aerosol: 84 μg/spray	**6-12 yrs:** 2 inhalations bid.
	BECONASE, VANCENASE		Nasal Aerosol: 42 μg/spray	**6-12 yrs:** 1 inhalation in each nostril tid.
	BECONASE AQ, VANCENASE AQ		Nasal Spray: 0.042% (42 μg/spray)	**6-12 yrs:** 1 - 2 inhalations in each nostril bid.
	VANCENASE AQ 84 MCG		Nasal Spray: 0.084% (84 μg/spray)	**6-12 yrs:** 1 or 2 inhalations in each nostril bid.
Benzalkonium Chloride	ZEPHIRAN CHLORIDE	Antiseptic	Solution & Spray: 1:750	Apply liberally to skin prn.

Generic	Brand	Category	Form/Strength	Dosage
Benzocaine	BABY ORAJEL, BABY ANBESOL	Local Anesthetic (Oral)	Gel: 7.5%	Over 4 mos: Apply a small pea-size amount with fingertip or cotton applicator to the affected mouth area up to qid.
	ANBESOL MAXIMUM STRENGTH	Local Anesthetic (Oral)	Liquid & Gel: 20%	Over 2 yrs: Apply to the affected area on or within the mouth up to qid.
	AMERICAINE OTIC	Local Anesthetic (Topical)	Otic Solution: 20%	Over 1 yr: Instill 4 - 5 drops into the ear canal, then insert a cotton pledget into the meatus. May repeat q 1 - 2 h if necessary.
	AMERICAINE	Local Anesthetic (Topical)	Lubricant Gel: 20%	Over 1 yr: Apply evenly to exterior of tube or instrument prior to use.
			Spray: 20%	Over 2 yrs: Apply liberally to affected areas not more than tid or qid.
Benzonatate	TESSALON	Antitussive	Cpsl: 100 mg	Over 10 yrs: 100 mg tid po.
Betamethasone Dipropionate, Regular	DIPROSONE, MAXIVATE	Corticosteroid	Cream & Oint: 0.05% Lotion: 0.05%	Apply a thin film to affected areas once daily. Massage a few drops into affected areas bid.
	DIPROSONE		Topical Aerosol: 0.1%	Apply sparingly to affected skin areas tid.
Betamethasone Valerate	VALISONE	Corticosteroid	Cream & Oint: 0.1%	Apply a thin film to affected areas 1 - 3 times daily.
			Lotion: 0.1%	Massage a few drops into affected areas bid.
	VALISONE REDUCED STRENGTH		Cream: 0.01%	Apply a thin film to affected areas 1 - 3 times daily.
Bisacodyl	DULCOLAX, FLEET LAXATIVE	Stimulant Laxative	Tab: 5 mg	6-12 yrs: 5 mg once daily po.
			Rectal Suppos: 10 mg	6-12 yrs: Insert 1/2 suppository (5 mg) rectally once daily.
	CORRECTOL		Cplt & Tab: 5 mg	6-12 yrs: 5 mg once daily po.
	FLEET BISACODYL ENEMA		Rectal Suspension: 10 mg/30 mL	6-12 yrs: Administer 15 mL rectally in a single daily dose.

GENERIC NAME	COMMON TRADE NAMES	THERAPEUTIC CATEGORY	PREPARATIONS	COMMON PEDIATRIC DOSAGE
Bismuth Subsalicylate	PEPTO-BISMOL	Antidiarrheal	Susp: 262 mg/15 mL Chewable Tab: 262 mg Cplt: 262 mg	**Under 3 yrs (dose po according to body weight)**: Repeat q 4 h prn to a maximum of 6 doses per day. **14-18 lbs**: 2.5 mL of Suspension. **18-28 lbs**: 5 mL of Suspension. **3-6 yrs**: 5 mL or 1/3 tab or cplt po. **6-9 yrs**: 10 mL or 2/3 tab or cplt po. **9-12 yrs**: 15 mL or 1 tab or cplt po. **Over 12 yrs**: 30 mL or 2 tabs or cplts po. Repeat above dose q 1/2 - 1 h prn to a maximum of 8 doses per day.
	PEPTO-BISMOL MAXIMUM STRENGTH		Susp: 525 mg/15 mL	**3-6 yrs**: 5 mL po. **6-9 yrs**: 10 mL po. **9-12 yrs**: 15 mL po. Repeat above dose q 1 h prn to a maximum of 4 doses per day.
Brompheniramine Maleate	DIMETAPP ALLERGY	Antihistamine	Tab: 4 mg	**6-12 yrs**: 2 mg q 4 - 6 h po.
Budesonide	RHINOCORT	Corticosteroid	Aerosol: 32 µg/spray	**Over 6 yrs**: 256 µg daily, given as either 2 sprays in each nostril in the morning and evening or 4 sprays in each nostril in the morning.
	PULMICORT TURBUHALER		Aerosol: 200 µg/spray	**Over 6 yrs**: 200 µg bid by oral inhalation.
Buprenorphine Hydrochloride (C-V)	BUPRENEX	Opioid Analgesic	Inj: 0.3 mg/mL	**2-12 yrs**: 2 - 6 µg/kg by deep IM or slow IV over at least 2 minutes) q 4 - 6 h.
Busulfan	MYLERAN	Antineoplastic	Tab: 2 mg	Daily dosage range is 4 - 8 mg po. Dosing on a weight basis is approximately 60 µg/kg daily or 1.8 mg/m² daily.
Butabarbital Sodium (C-III)	BUTISOL SODIUM	Sedative	Elixir: 30 mg/5 mL (7% alcohol) Tab: 15, 30, 50, 100 mg	**Preoperative Sedation**: 2 - 6 mg/kg/day po. Maximum: 100 mg.

Butamben Picrate	BUTESIN PICRATE	Local Anesthetic (Topical)	**Oint:** 1%	Spread thinly on painful or denuded lesions of the skin, if these are small. Apply a loose bandage to protect the clothing.
Calcitriol	ROCALTROL	Vitamin D Analog	**Cpsl:** 0.25, 0.5 µg	**Hypoparathyroidism (Over 6 yrs):** 0.25 µg daily po given in the AM. The dosage may be increased at 2 to 4 week intervals. Most patients respond to doses between 0.5 and 2 µg daily.
Calcium Carbonate	CHILDREN'S MYLANTA UPSET STOMACH RELIEF	Antacid	**Liquid:** 400 mg/5 mL **Chewable Tab:** 400 mg	**2-5 yrs (24-47 lbs):** 400 mg po up to tid. **6-11 yrs (48-95 lbs):** 800 mg po up to tid.
Calcium Glubionate	NEO-CALGLUCON	Calcium Supplement	**Syrup:** 1.8 g/5 mL (equal to 115 mg of calcium/5 mL)	**Dietary Supplement:** **Infants:** 5 mL 5 times daily po. **Under 4 yrs:** 10 mL tid po. **Over 4 yrs:** 15 mL tid po.
Calcium Polycarbophil	MITROLAN	Bulk Laxative	**Chewable Tab:** 500 mg	**3-6 yrs:** Chew and swallow 1 tab bid. **6-12 yrs:** Chew and swallow 1 tab tid. A full glass of liquid (8 oz.) should be taken with each dose indicated above.
	FIBERCON, KONSYL		**Tab:** 625 mg	**6-12 yrs:** Swallow 1 tab 1 - 4 times daily. A full glass of liquid (8 oz.) should be taken with each dose.
	FIBERALL		**Chewable Tab:** 1000 mg	**6-12 yrs:** Chew and swallow 1/2 tab 1 - 4 times daily. A full glass of liquid (8 oz.) should be taken with each dose.
Calcium Undecylenate	CRUEX (Original)	Antifungal	**Powder:** 10%	**Over 2 yrs:** Apply a thin layer onto the affected areas bid. AM and PM.
	CALDESENE	Diaper Rash Product	**Powder:** 10%	After cleaning and throughly drying the skin, smooth powder directly onto baby's skin.

GENERIC NAME	COMMON TRADE NAMES	THERAPEUTIC CATEGORY	PREPARATIONS	COMMON PEDIATRIC DOSAGE
Capsaicin	ZOSTRIX	Analgesic, Topical	Cream: 0.025%	**Over 2 yrs:** Apply to affected area tid or qid.
	ZOSTRIX-HP		Cream: 0.075%	**Over 2 yrs:** Apply to affected area tid or qid.
Carbamazepine	TEGRETOL	Antiepileptic	Susp: 100 mg/5 mL Chewable Tab: 100 mg Tab: 200 mg	**Under 6 yrs (Initial):** 10 - 20 mg/kg/day qid (Susp) or tid or qid (Tabs) po. Increase at weekly intervals to achieve optimal clinical response using a tid or qid regimen. **Under 6 yrs (Maintenance):** Usually, optimal clinical response occurs at daily doses below 35 mg/kg po.
	TEGRETOL-XR		Extended-Rel. Tab: 100, 200, 400 mg	**6-12 yrs (Initial):** 50 mg qid (Susp) or 100 mg bid (Tabs or XR Tabs) po. Increase at weekly intervals by adding up to 100 mg per day using a tid or qid regimen (Susp or Tabs) or a bid regimen (XR Tabs) until the optimal response is obtained. Maximum: 1000 mg per day. **6-12 yrs (Maintenance):** Adjust dose to the minimum effective level, usually 400 - 800 mg daily po.
Carbamide Peroxide	GLY-OXIDE	Antiseptic	Liquid: 10%	**Over 2 yrs:** Apply several drops onto the affected mouth area; spit out after 2 mins. Use up to qid pc & hs.
Castor Oil (Plain)		Stimulant Laxative	Liquid: (pure)	**6-12 yrs:** 5 - 10 mL po.
Castor Oil, Emulsified	NEOLOID	Stimulant Laxative	Liquid: 36.4% w/w	**Infants:** 2.5 - 7.5 mL po. **Children:** Adjust between the infant dose and and the adult dose of 30 - 60 mL po.
	FLEET FLAVORED CASTOR OIL EMULSION		Liquid: 67% v/v (10 mL of castor oil/15 mL)	**1-2 yrs:** 5 mL po. **2-12 yrs:** 15 mL po.

34

Castor Oil, Flavored	PURGE	Stimulant Laxative	Liquid: 95% w/w	Infants: 5 - 10 mL po. Children: Adjust between the infant dose and and the adult dose of 30 - 60 mL po.
Cefaclor	CECLOR	Antibacterial	Powd for Susp (per 5 mL): 125, 187, 250, 375 mg Cpsl: 250, 500 mg	Usual Dosage: 20 mg/kg/day in divided doses q 8 h po. More Serious Infections and Otitis Media: 40 mg/kg/day in divided doses q 8 h po. Maximum: 1 g/day.
Cefadroxil Monohydrate	DURICEF	Antibacterial	Powd for Susp (per 5 mL): 125, 250, 500 mg Cpsl: 500 mg	Urinary Tract and Skin and Skin Structure Infections: 30 mg/kg/day po in divided doses q 12 h. Pharyngitis, Tonsillitis, and Impetigo: 30 mg/kg/day po in a single dose or in equally divided doses q 12 h.
Cefazolin Sodium	ANCEF, KEFZOL	Antibacterial	Powd for Inj: 500, 1000 mg	Mild to Moderately Severe Infections (Over 1 mo): 25 - 50 mg/kg/day IM or IV in divided doses q 6 - 8 h. Severe Infections (Over 1 mo): 100 mg/kg/day IM or IV in divided doses q 6 - 8 h.
Cefdinir	OMNICEF	Antibacterial	Powd for Susp: 125 mg/5 mL Cpsl: 300 mg	Acute Bacterial Otitis Media & Acute Maxillary Sinusitis (6 mos - 12 yrs): 7 mg/kg q 12 h po or 14 mg/kg q 24 h po for 10 days. Skin and Skin Structure Infections, Uncompl. (6 mos - 12 yrs): 7 mg/kg q 12 h po for 10 days. Pharyngitis / Tonsillitis (6 mos - 12 yrs): 7 mg/kg q 12 h po for 5 - 10 days or 14 mg/kg q 24 h po for 10 days.
Cefixime	SUPRAX	Antibacterial	Powd for Susp: 100 mg/5 mL Tab: 200, 400 mg	Over 6 mos: 8 mg/kg/day po as a single daily dose or as 4 mg/kg q 12 h po.

GENERIC NAME	COMMON TRADE NAMES	THERAPEUTIC CATEGORY	PREPARATIONS	COMMON PEDIATRIC DOSAGE
Cefotaxime Sodium	CLAFORAN	Antibacterial	**Powd for Inj:** 0.5 1, 2 g **Inj (per 50 mL):** 1, 2 g	**Birth - 1 wk:** 50 mg/kg IV q 12 h. **1-4 wks:** 50 mg/kg IV q 8 h. **1 mo - 12 yrs:** **Under 50 kg:** 50 - 180 mg/kg/day IM or IV in equally divided doses q 4 - 6 h (Maximum: 12 g per day). **Over 50 kg:** Use adult dosages.
Cefoxitin Sodium	MEFOXIN	Antibacterial	**Powd for Inj:** 1, 2 g **Inj (per 50 mL):** 1, 2 g	**Over 3 mos:** 80 - 160 mg/kg/day IV in divided doses q 4 - 6 h. Maximum: 8 - 12 g/day.
Cefpodoxime Proxetil	VANTIN	Antibacterial	**Powd for Susp (per 5 mL):** 50, 100 mg **Tab:** 100, 200 mg	**Pharyngitis & Tonsillitis (5 mos - 12 yrs):** 5 mg/kg q 12 h po for 5 - 10 days. Maximum: 200 mg/day. **Acute Otitis Media (5 mos - 12 yrs):** 5 mg/kg q 12 h po for 10 days or 10 mg/kg q 24 h po for 10 days. Maximum: 400 mg/day.
Cefprozil	CEFZIL	Antibacterial	**Powd for Susp (per 5 mL):** 125, 250 mg **Tab:** 250, 500 mg	**Otitis Media (6 mos - 12 yrs):** 15 mg/kg q 12 h po for 10 days. **Acute Sinusitis (6 mos - 12 yrs):** 7.5 - 15 mg/kg q 12 h po for 10 days. **Pharyngitis/Tonsillitis (2 - 12 yrs):** 7.5 mg/kg q 12 h po for at least 10 days. **Skin & Skin Structure Infections (2 - 12 yrs):** 20 mg/kg q 24 h po for 10 days.
Ceftazidime	FORTAZ, TAZIDIME	Antibacterial	**Powd for Inj:** 0.5, 1, 2 g	**Birth - 4 wks:** 30 mg/kg q 12 h IV. **1 mo - 12 yrs:** 30 - 50 mg/kg q 8 h IV. Maximum: 6 g/day.
Ceftazidime Sodium	FORTAZ	Antibacterial	**Inj (per 50 mL):** 1, 2 g	Same dosages as for FORTAZ above.
Ceftibuten	CEDAX	Antibacterial	**Powd for Susp (per 5 mL):** 90, 180 mg **Cpsl:** 400 mg	9 mg/kg once daily po at least 2 h before or 1 h after a meal for 10 days. Maximum daily dose is 400 mg.

Drug	Brand	Class	Forms	Dosage
Ceftizoxime Sodium	CEFIZOX	Antibacterial	**Inj (per 20, 50, or 100 mL):** 1, 2 g	**Over 6 mos:** 50 mg/kg q 6 - 8 h IM or IV. Maximum: 6 g/day.
Ceftriaxone Sodium	ROCEPHIN	Antibacterial	**Powd for Inj:** 250, 500 mg; 1, 2 g	**Usual Dosage:** 50 - 75 mg/kg/day in divided doses q 12 h IM or IV. Maximum: 2 g/day. **Meningitis:** 100 mg/kg/day in divided doses q 12 h IM or IV, with or without a loading dose of 75 mg/kg.
Cefuroxime Axetil	CEFTIN	Antibacterial	**Powd for Susp (per 5 mL):** 125, 250 mg **Tab:** 125, 250, 500 mg	**Pharyngitis/Tonsillitis (3 mos - 12 yrs):** 10 mg/kg bid po for 10 days. Maximum: 500 mg. **Acute Otitis Media & Impetigo (3 mos - 12 yrs):** 15 mg/kg bid po for 10 days. Maximum: 1000 mg. **Children Who Can Swallow Tablets:** **Pharyngitis/Tonsillitis:** 125 mg bid po for 10 days. **Acute Otitis Media:** 250 mg bid po for 10 days.
Cefuroxime Sodium	KEFUROX, ZINACEF	Antibacterial	**Powd for Inj:** 0.75, 1.5 g	**Most Infections (Over 3 mos):** 50 - 100 mg/kg/day in equally divided doses q 6 - 8 h IM or IV. Maximum: 4.5 g/day. **Bone & Joint Infections (Over 3 mos):** 150 mg/kg/day in equally divided doses q 8 h IM or IV. Maximum: 4.5 g/day. **Meningitis (Over 3 mos):** 200 - 240 mg/kg/day in divided doses q 6 - 8 h IM or IV.
Cephalexin	KEFLEX	Antibacterial	**Powd for Susp (Drops):** 100 mg/mL **Powd for Susp (per 5 mL):** 125, 250 mg **Cpsl:** 250, 500 mg	**Usual Dosage:** 25 - 50 mg/kg/day in divided doses q 6 h po. **Streptococcal Pharyngitis (Over 1 yr) and Skin and Skin Structure Infections:** 25 - 50 mg/kg daily in divided doses q 12 h po. In severe infections, the dosage may be doubled. **Otitis Media:** 75 - 100 mg/kg/day in 4 divided doses po.

GENERIC NAME	COMMON TRADE NAMES	THERAPEUTIC CATEGORY	PREPARATIONS	COMMON PEDIATRIC DOSAGE
Cephapirin Sodium	CEFADYL	Antibacterial	Powd for Inj: 1 g	40 - 80 mg/kg/day in 4 equally divided doses IV or IM.
Cephradine	VELOSEF	Antibacterial	Powd for Susp (per 5 mL): 125, 250, 500 mg Cpsl: 250, 500 mg	**Over 9 mos:** 25 - 50 mg/kg/day in equally divided doses q 6 - 12 h po. **Otitis Media due to** *H. influenzae***:** 75 - 100 mg/kg/day in equally divided doses q 6 - 12 h po. Maximum: 4 g/day.
			Powd for Inj: 250, 500 mg; 1, 2 g	**Over 1 mo:** 50 - 100 mg/kg/day in 4 equally divided doses IM or IV.
Cetirizine Hydrochloride	ZYRTEC	Antihistamine	Syrup: 5 mg/5 mL Tab: 5, 10 mg	**Over 6 yrs:** 5 - 10 mg once daily po depending on the severity of symptoms.
Chloral Hydrate (C-IV)		Sedative - Hypnotic	Syrup: 500 mg/5 mL Cpsl: 500 mg	**Sedation:** 25 mg/kg q 8 h po. **Hypnosis:** 50 mg/kg po.
Chloramphenicol		Antibacterial	Cpsl: 250 mg	**Under 2 wks:** 25 mg/kg/day in equally divided doses q 6 h po. **Over 2 wks:** 50 mg/kg/day in equally divided doses q 6 h po.
	CHLOROPTIC		Ophth Solution: 0.5%	1 - 2 drops into the affected eye(s) 4 - 6 times daily for the first 72 hours, depending on the severity of the condition. Intervals between doses may be increased after the first 2 days.
	CHLOROPTIC S.O.P.		Ophth Oint: 1%	Place a small amount of ointment in the affected eye(s) q 3 h, or more often if required, day & night for he first 48 h; then intervals between doses may be increased after the first 2 days.

38

Drug	Classification	Form	Dosage
Chloramphenicol Sodium Succinate	Antibacterial	**Powd for Inj:** 100 mg/mL (when reconstituted)	**Under 2 wks:** 25 mg/kg/day in equally divided doses q 6 h IV. **Over 2 wks:** 50 mg/kg/day in equally divided doses q 6 h IV.
Chlordiazepoxide Hydrochloride (C-IV) LIBRIUM	Antianxiety Agent	**Cpsl:** 5, 10, 25 mg	**Over 6 yrs:** Usually 5 mg bid to qid po; may be increased in some to 10 mg bid or tid.
Chloroquine Hydrochloride ARALEN HCL	Antimalarial	**Inj:** 50 mg salt (= to 40 mg of chloroquine base)/mL	5 mg/kg of chloroquine base IM initially; repeat in 6 h if necessary. Maximum: 10 mg/kg of chloroquine base per 24 hours.
Chloroquine Phosphate ARALEN PHOSPHATE	Antimalarial	**Tab:** 500 mg salt (= to 300 mg of chloroquine base)	**Suppression:** 5 mg/kg of chloroquine base once weekly po. on the same day each week, but not to exceed the adult dose of 300 mg of base. **Acute Attacks:** Initially, 10 mg/kg of chloroquine base po. followed by 5 mg/kg chloroquine base, 6 h later, 5 mg/kg 18 h after the 2nd dose. A 4th dose of 5 mg/kg should be given 24 h after the 3rd dose.
Chlorothiazide DIURIL	Diuretic	**Susp:** 250 mg/5 mL (0.5% alcohol) **Tab:** 250, 500 mg	Usually 10 mg/lb/day po in 2 divided doses. Infants under 6 months may require up to 15 mg/lb/day in 2 doses. On this basis: **Birth - 2 yrs:** 125 - 375 mg daily po in 2 doses (of the Suspension). **2-12 yrs:** 375 - 1000 mg daily po in 2 doses.
Chlorpheniramine Maleate PEDIACARE ALLERGY FORMULA	Antihistamine	**Liquid:** 1 mg/5 mL	**2-3 yrs:** 5 mL (1 mg) q 4 - 6 h po. **4-5 yrs:** 7.5 mL (1.5 mg) q 4 - 6 h po. **6-8 yrs:** 10 mL (2 mg) q 4 - 6 h po. **9-10 yrs:** 12.5 mL (2.5 mg) q 4 - 6 h po. **11-12 yrs:** 15 mL (3 mg) q 4 - 6 h po.

[Continued on the next page]

39

GENERIC NAME	COMMON TRADE NAMES	THERAPEUTIC CATEGORY	PREPARATIONS	COMMON PEDIATRIC DOSAGE
Chlorpheniramine Maleate [Continued]	CHLOR-TRIMETON ALLERGY 4 HOUR		**Syrup:** 2 mg/5 mL (7% alcohol) **Tab:** 4 mg	**2-5 yrs:** 2.5 mL (1 mg) q 4 - 6 h po. **6-12 yrs:** 5 mL (2 mg) q 4 - 6 h po.
			Inj: 10 mg/mL	0.35 mg/kg/day in divided doses q 6 h IM or SC.
Chlorpromazine	THORAZINE	Antiemetic, Antipsychotic	**Suppos:** 25, 100 mg	**Emesis (Over 6 mos):** 0.5 mg/lb q 6 - 8 h rectally, prn. **Severe Behavioral Problems (Outpatients, Over 6 mos):** 0.5 mg/lb q 6 - 8 h rectally, prn.
Chlorpromazine Hydrochloride	THORAZINE	Antipsychotic, Antiemetic	**Syrup:** 10 mg/5 mL **Liquid Conc:** 30, 100 mg/mL **Tab:** 10, 25, 50, 100, 200 mg	**Severe Behavioral Problems (Over 6 mos old):** **Outpatients:** Usually 0.25 mg/lb q 4 - 6 h po; increase dosage gradually as required. **Hospitalized Patients:** 50 - 100 mg daily po, and in older children, 200 mg or more, may be necessary. **Emesis (Over 6 mos):** 0.25 mg/lb q 4 - 6 h po. **Presurgical Apprehension:** 0.25 mg po 2 - 3 h before the operation.
			Inj: 25 mg/mL	**Severe Behavioral Problems (Over 6 mos old):** **Outpatients:** Usually 0.25 mg/lb q 6 - 8 h IM; increase dosage gradually as required. **Hospitalized Patients:** Start with low doses and increase dosage gradually. Maximum IM dosage: 40 mg/day (up to 5 yrs or 50 lbs); 75 mg/day (5 to 12 yrs or 50 to 100 lbs) except in unmanageable cases. **Emesis (Over 6 mos):** 0.25 mg/lb q 6 - 8 h IM. Maximum IM dosage: 40 mg/day (up to 5 yrs or 50 lbs); 75 mg/day (5 to 12 yrs or 50 to 100 lbs) except in severe cases.

40

Drug	Brand	Class	Form	Dosage
Ciclopirox Olamine	LOPROX	Antifungal	Cream & Lotion: 1%	**Over 10 yrs:** Gently massage into affected and surrounding skin areas bid, in the AM and PM.
Ciprofloxacin Hydrochloride	CILOXAN	Antibacterial	Ophth Solution: 0.3% (as the base)	**Corneal Ulcers (Over 1 yr):** 2 drops in the affected eye(s) q 15 min for the 1st 6 hours, then 2 drops q 30 min for the rest of the 1st day. Second day: 2 drops q 1 h; 3rd to 14th day: 2 drops q 4 h. **Conjunctivitis (Over 1 yr):** 1 - 2 drops in the affected eye(s) q 2 h while awake for 2 days, then 1 - 2 drops q 4 h while awake for the next 5 days.
			Ophth Oint: 0.3% (as the base)	**Over 2 yrs:** Place 1/2 in strip into conjunctival sac tid for 2 days, then bid for 5 days.
Cisatracurium Besylate	NIMBEX	Neuromuscular Blocker	Inj (per mL): 2, 10 mg	**2-12 yrs:** Initial dose is 0.10 mg/kg IV (over 5 - 10 sec).
Clarithromycin	BIAXIN	Antibacterial	Gran for Susp (per 5 mL): 125, 250 mg Tab: 250, 500 mg	**Usual Dosage:** 7.5 mg/kg po q 12 h for 10 days. Maximum: 500 mg/day. Dosing Guidelines by body weight: **9 kg (20 lbs):** 62.5 mg po q 12 h. **17 kg (37 lbs):** 125 mg po q 12 h. **25 kg (55 lbs):** 187.5 mg po q 12 h. **33 kg (73 lbs):** 250 mg po q 12 h. *Mycobacterium avium* **complex:** 7.5 mg/kg po bid, up to 500 mg bid.

For Nausea & Vomiting During Surgery:
IM: 0.125 mg/lb. Repeat in 30 minutes if necessary and no hypotension occurs.
IV: 1 mg/fractional injection at 2-minute intervals and not exceeding IM dosage. Always dilute to 1 mg/mL with saline.
Presurgical Apprehension: 0.25 mg IM 1 - 2 h before the operation.

GENERIC NAME	COMMON TRADE NAMES	THERAPEUTIC CATEGORY	PREPARATIONS	COMMON PEDIATRIC DOSAGE
Clemastine Fumarate	TAVIST	Antihistamine	**Syrup:** 0.67 mg/5 mL (5.5% alcohol)	**Allergic Rhinitis (6-12 yrs):** 5 mL (0.5 mg of clemastine base) bid po. **Urticaria and Angioedema (6-12 yrs):** 10 mL (1 mg of clemastine base) bid po.
Clindamycin Hydrochloride	CLEOCIN HCL	Antibacterial	**Cpsl:** 75, 150, 300 mg	**Serious Infections:** 8 - 16 mg/kg/day po, divided into 3 or 4 equal doses. **More Severe Infections:** 16 - 20 mg/kg/day po, divided into 3 or 4 equal doses.
Clindamycin Palmitate Hydrochloride	CLEOCIN PEDIATRIC	Antibacterial	**Granules for Susp:** 75 mg/5 mL	**Serious Infections:** 8 - 12 mg/kg/day po, divided into 3 or 4 equal doses. **Severe Infections:** 13 - 16 mg/kg/day po, divided into 3 or 4 equal doses. **More Severe Infections:** 17 - 25 mg/kg/day po, divided into 3 or 4 equal doses. **Under 10 kg:** 2.5 mL (37.5 mg) tid po should be considered the minimum dose.
Clindamycin Phosphate	CLEOCIN PHOSPHATE	Antibacterial	**Inj:** 150 mg/mL	**Under 1 mo:** 15 - 20 mg/kg/day IV in 3 - 4 equal doses. **Over 1 mo:** 20 - 40 mg/kg/day IV or IM in 3 or 4 equal doses.
Clioquinol	VIOFORM	Antifungal	**Cream & Oint:** 3%	**Over 2 yrs:** Apply to the affected area bid or tid.
Clomipramine Hydrochloride	ANAFRANIL	Drug for Obsessive-Compulsive Disorder	**Cpsl:** 25, 50, 75 mg	**Over 10 yrs:** Initially, 25 mg daily po; this should be gradually increased (in divided doses with meals) during the first 2 weeks, as tolerated, up to a daily maximum of 3 mg/kg or 100 mg, whichever is smaller. Thereafter, the dosage may be increased gradually over the next several weeks up to a daily maximum of 3 mg/kg or 200 mg, whichever is smaller.

Drug	Brand	Class	Form	Dosage
Clonazepam (C-IV)	KLONOPIN	Antiepileptic	Tab: 0.5, 1, 2 mg	**Up to 10 yrs or 30 kg:** 0.01 - 0.03 mg/kg/day po in 2 or 3 divided doses. Dosage should be increased by no more than 0.25 - 0.5 mg every third day until a daily maintenance dose of 0.1 - 0.2 mg/kg has been reached.
Clorazepate Dipotassium (C-IV)	TRANXENE-T TAB	Antiepileptic	Tab: 3.75, 7.5, 15 mg	**9-12 yrs:** 3.75 - 7.5 mg bid po. Dosage should be increased no more than 7.5 mg every week and should not exceed 60 mg per day.
Clotrimazole	MYCELEX	Antifungal	Troches: 10 mg	**Over 3 yrs:** Slowly dissolve 1 in the mouth 5 times daily for 14 consecutive days.
	LOTRIMIN AF		Cream, Lotion & Solution: 1%	Gently massage into affected and surrounding skin areas bid, AM and PM.
	MYCELEX		Cream & Solution: 1%	Gently massage into affected and surrounding skin areas bid, AM and PM.
	CRUEX, DESENEX		Cream: 1%	**Over 2 yrs:** Apply a thin layer to the affected areas bid, AM and PM.
Cloxacillin Sodium		Antibacterial	Powd for Solution: 125 mg/5 mL Cpsl: 250, 500 mg	**Mild to Moderate Infections:** **Under 20 kg:** 50 mg/kg/day po in equally divided doses q 6 h. **Over 20 kg:** 250 mg q 6 h po. **Severe Infections:** **Under 20 kg:** 100 mg/kg/day po in equally divided doses q 6 h. **Over 20 kg:** 500 mg q 6 h po.
Codeine Phosphate (C-II)		Opioid Analgesic	Inj (per mL): 30, 60 mg	**Over 1 yr:** 0.5 mg/kg q 4 - 6 h SC or IM.
Codeine Sulfate (C-II)		Opioid Analgesic, Antitussive	Tab: 15, 30, 60 mg	**Analgesic (Over 1 yr):** 0.5 mg/kg q 4 - 6 h po. **Antitussive:** 0.2 mg/kg q 4 h po. **2-6 yrs:** 2.5 - 5 mg q 4 - 6 h po. **6-12 yrs:** 5 - 10 mg q 4 - 6 h po.

43

GENERIC NAME	COMMON TRADE NAMES	THERAPEUTIC CATEGORY	PREPARATIONS	COMMON PEDIATRIC DOSAGE
Colfosceril Palmitate	EXOSURF NEONATAL	Lung Surfactant	Powd for Susp: 108 mg	**Prophylactic Treatment:** 5 mL/kg intratracheally as soon as possible after birth. Administer the 2nd and 3rd doses approximately 12 and 24 h later to all infants who remain on mechanical ventilation at these times. **Rescue Treatment:** Administer two 5 mL/kg doses intratracheally. The 2nd dose is given 12 h after the 1st dose, provided the infant remains on mechanical ventilation.
Colistimethate Sodium	COLY-MYCIN M PARENTERAL	Antibacterial	**Powd for Inj:** 150 mg (= to colistin base)	2.5 - 5.0 mg/kg per day in 2 - 4 divided doses IV or IM.
Cromolyn Sodium	INTAL	Antiasthmatic	**Solution (for Nebulization):** 20 mg/2 mL **Inhaler:** 800 µg/spray	**Over 2 yrs:** 20 mg qid nebulized. **Over 5 yrs:** 2 sprays inhaled qid.
	GASTROCROM	Antiallergic	**Cpsl:** 100 mg **Conc. Solution:** 100 mg/5 mL	**2-12 yrs:** 100 mg qid po, 30 minutes ac & hs.
	CROLOM	Antiallergic	**Ophth Solution:** 4%	**Over 4 yrs:** 1 or 2 drops in each eye 4 - 6 times daily at regular intervals.
	NASALCROM	Antiallergic	**Nasal Solution:** 40 mg/mL (4%)	**Over 6 yrs:** 1 spray in each nostril tid - qid (q 4 - 6 h). If necessary, may use up to 6 times daily.
Cyclizine Hydrochloride	MAREZINE	Antiemetic	**Tab:** 50 mg	**6-12 yrs:** 25 mg q 6 - 8 h po.

44

Cyclopentolate Hydrochloride	CYCLOGYL	Mydriatic - Cycloplegic	Ophth Solution: 0.5, 1, 2%	**Infants:** 1 drop of 0.5% solution into each eye. Compress inner canthus for 2 - 3 mins to reduce absorption. Observe patient closely for at least 30 min following instillation. **Older Children:** 1 or 2 drops into each eye of 0.5%, 1%, or 2% solution. Compress inner canthus for 1 min to reduce absorption. Follow in 5 - 10 mins with a second application of 0.5% or 1% solution.
Cyclophosphamide	CYTOXAN	Antineoplastic	Tab: 25, 50 mg Powd for Inj: 100, 200, 500 mg: 1, 2 g	**Malignant Disease:** 1 - 5 mg/kg/day po. **Biopsy Proven "Minimal Change" Nephrotic Syndrome:** 2.5 - 3.0 mg/kg daily po for 60 to 90 days. **Malignant Disease:** 40 - 50 mg/kg IV in divided doses over a period of 2 - 5 days; or 10 - 15 mg/kg IV q 7 - 10 days; or 3 - 5 mg/kg IV twice weekly.
Cyproheptadine Hydrochloride	PERIACTIN	Antihistamine, Antipruritic	Syrup: 2 mg/5 mL (5% alcohol) Tab: 4 mg	0.25 mg/kg/day po in divided doses q 6 - 8 h or by age: **2-6 yrs:** 2 mg bid or tid po. **7-14 yrs:** 4 mg bid or tid po.
Cytarabine	CYTOSAR-U	Antineoplastic	Powd for Inj: 100, 500 mg: 1, 2 g	100 mg/m²/day by continuous IV infusion (Days 1 - 7) or 100 mg/m² IV q 12 h (Days 1 - 7).
Dactinomycin	COSMEGEN	Antineoplastic	Powd for Inj: 0.5 mg	**Over 12 mos:** 15 µg/kg/day IV for 5 days. An alternative schedule is a total dose of 2500 µg/m² IV over a 1 week period.
Dantrolene Sodium	DANTRIUM	Skeletal Muscle Relaxant	Cpsl: 25, 50, 100 mg	**Chronic Spasticity:** Initially 0.5 mg/kg once daily po for 7 days; then 0.5 mg/kg tid for 7 days; then 1.0 mg/kg tid for 7 days; then 2 mg/kg tid. Therapy in some patients may require qid dosing. Max: 100 mg qid po.

[Continued on the next page]

45

GENERIC NAME	COMMON TRADE NAMES	THERAPEUTIC CATEGORY	PREPARATIONS	COMMON PEDIATRIC DOSAGE
Dantrolene Sodium [Continued]	DANTRIUM INTRAVENOUS		Powd for Inj: 20 mg	**Malignant Hyperthermia:** **Acute Therapy:** Administer by continuous rapid IV push beginning at a minimum dose of 1 mg/kg, and continuing until the symptoms subside or the max. cumulative dose of 10 mg/kg has been reached. **Preoperatively:** 2.5 mg/kg IV starting approx. 1.25 hours before anticipated anesthesia and infused over 1 h. **Post Crisis Follow Up:** Individualize, starting with 1 mg/kg IV.
Demeclocycline Hydrochloride	DECLOMYCIN	Antibacterial	Tab: 150, 300 mg	Over 8 yrs: 3 - 6 mg/lb/day po divided into 2 to 4 doses po.
Desmopressin Acetate	DDAVP NASAL SPRAY	Posterior Pituitary Hormone, Anti-Enuretic Agent	Nasal Spray: 0.1 mg/mL (delivers 0.1 mL (10 μg) per spray)	Central Cranial Diabetes Insipidus (Over 3 mos): 0.05 - 0.3 mL daily intranasally, as a single dose or in 2 divided doses.
	DDAVP RHINAL TUBE		Nasal Solution: 0.1 mg/mL (with rhinal tube applicators)	Primary Nocturnal Enuresis (Over 6 yrs): 0.2 mL intranasally hs. Dosage adjustment up to 0.4 mL may be made if necessary.
	DDAVP TABLETS		Tab: 0.1, 0.2 mg	Central Cranial Diabetes Insipidus: Initially, 0.05 mg bid po. Dosage adjustments may be made such that the total daily dosage is in the range of 0.1 - 1.2 mg divided tid or bid.
	DDAVP INJECTION		Inj: 4.0 μg/mL	Hemophilia A and von Willebrand's Disease (Type I): 0.3 μg/kg diluted in sterile saline (50 mL if over 10 kg; 10 mL if ≤ 10 kg); infuse IV slowly over 15 - 30 minutes. If used preop., give 30 min. prior to procedure.
	STIMATE	Posterior Pituitary Hormone	Nasal Spray: 1.5 mg/mL (delivers 0.1 mL (150 μg) per spray)	Hemophilia A and von Willebrand's Disease (Type I) (Over 11 mos): 1 spray per nostril (total of 300 μg) in patients weighing ≥ 50 kg; 1 spray in nostril only in patients weighing < 50 kg.

Desonide	TRIDESILON	Corticosteroid	Cream & Oint: 0.05%	Apply to the affected areas bid to qid.
Desoximetasone	TOPICORT	Corticosteroid	Cream: 0.05, 0.25% Gel: 0.05%	Apply a thin film to the affected areas bid. Rub in gently.
			Oint: 0.25%	**Over 10 yrs:** Apply a thin film to the affected areas bid. Rub in gently.
l-Desoxyephedrine	VICKS VAPOR INHALER	Nasal Decongestant	Inhaler: 50 mg	**6-12 yrs:** 1 inhalation in each nostril not more often than q 2 h.
Dexamethasone	DECADRON	Corticosteroid	Elixir: 0.5 mg/5 mL (5% alcohol) Tab: 0.5, 0.75, 4 mg	Initial dosage varies from 0.75 - 9 mg daily po, depending on the disease being treated. This should be maintained or adjusted until the patient's response is satisfactory.
Dexamethasone Sodium Phosphate	DEXACORT	Corticosteroid	Oral Inhaler (RESPIHALER): 100 μg/spray	**6-12 yrs:** 2 inhalations tid or qid. Maximum: 8 inhalations/day.
			Nasal Aerosol (TURBINAIRE): 100 μg/spray	**6-12 yrs:** 1 - 2 sprays in each nostril bid. Maximum: 8 sprays/day.
	DECADRON PHOSPHATE		Inj: 4 mg/mL	**IV and IM Inj:** Initial dosage varies from 0.5 - 9 mg daily depending on the disease being treated. This dosage should be maintained or adjusted until the patient's response is satisfactory.
			Inj: 24 mg/mL [for IV use only]	**Intra-articular, Intralesional, and Soft Tissue Injection:** Varies from 0.2 - 6 mg given from once q 3 - 5 days to once q 2 - 3 weeks.
			Topical Cream: 0.1%	Apply a thin film to affected area tid or qid.
Dexchlorpheniramine Maleate	POLARAMINE	Antihistamine	Syrup: 2 mg/5 mL (6% alcohol)	**2-5 yrs:** 1.25 mL (0.5 mg) q 4 - 6 h po. **6-11 yrs:** 2.5 mL (1 mg) q 4 - 6 h po.
			Tab: 2 mg	**2-5 yrs:** 0.5 mg q 4 - 6 h po. **6-11 yrs:** 1 mg q 4 - 6 h po.
			Repeat Action Tab: 4, 6 mg	**6-12 yrs:** One 4 mg tablet once daily po.

47

GENERIC NAME	COMMON TRADE NAMES	THERAPEUTIC CATEGORY	PREPARATIONS	COMMON PEDIATRIC DOSAGE
Dextroamphetamine Sulfate (C-II)	DEXEDRINE	CNS Stimulant	**Tab:** 5 mg **Sustained Rel. Cpsl:** 5, 10, 15 mg	**Attention Deficit Disorder:** **3-5 yrs:** Start with 2.5 mg daily po; daily dosage may be raised in increments of 2.5 mg at weekly intervals. **Over 6 yrs:** Double the above mg dosage schedule.
	DEXTROSTAT		**Tab:** 5, 10 mg	**Narcolepsy:** **6-12 yrs:** 5 mg daily po; daily dosage may be raised in increments of 5 mg weekly. Maximum: 60 mg daily. **Over 12 yrs:** Double the above mg dosage schedule. Maximum: 60 mg per day.
Dextromethorphan Hydrobromide	PERTUSSIN CS CHILDREN'S STRENGTH	Antitussive	**Syrup:** 3.5 mg/5 mL	**2-6 yrs:** 5 mL q 4 h po prn. **6-12 yrs:** 10 mL q 4 h po prn.
	BENYLIN PEDIATRIC COUGH SUPPRESSANT, ROBITUSSIN PEDIATRIC COUGH SUPPRESSANT		**Liquid:** 7.5 mg/5 mL	**2-6 yrs (24-47 lbs):** 5 mL q 6 - 8 h po. **6-12 yrs (48-95 lbs):** 10 mL q 6 - 8 h po.
	VICKS 44 COUGH RELIEF		**Liquid:** 10 mg/5 mL (alcohol 5%)	**6-11 yrs (48-95 lbs):** 7.5 mL q 6 - 8 h po. **12 yrs & older (over 95 lbs):** 15 mL q 6 - 8 h po.
	BENYLIN ADULT FORMULA, ROBITUSSIN MAXIMUM STRENGTH COUGH SUPPRESSANT		**Liquid:** 15 mg/5 mL	**2-6 yrs (24-47 lbs):** 2.5 mL q 6 - 8 h po. **6-12 yrs (48-95 lbs):** 5 mL q 6 - 8 h po.
	PERTUSSIN DM EXTRA STRENGTH		**Syrup:** 15 mg/5 mL	**6-12 yrs:** 5 mL q 6 - 8 h po.
	SUCRETS 4 HOUR COUGH SUPRESSANT		**Lozenge:** 15 mg	**6-12 yrs:** 1 lozenge po q 6 h prn.

48

Drug	Brand	Class	Forms/Strengths	Dosage
Dextromethorphan Polistirex	DELSYM	Antitussive	**Syrup:** equal to 30 mg dextromethorphan HBr/5 mL	2-6 yrs: 2.5 mL q 12 h po. 6-12 yrs: 5 mL q 12 h po.
Dextrothyroxine Sodium	CHOLOXIN	Hypolipidemic	**Tab:** 1, 2, 4 mg	Initial Dose: 0.05 mg/kg/day po. Maintenance dose: 0.1 mg/kg/day po.
Diazepam (C-IV)	VALIUM	Antianxiety Agent, Anticonvulsant, Skel. Muscle Relax.	**Tab:** 2, 5, 10 mg **Inj:** 5 mg/mL	Over 6 mos: 1 - 2.5 mg tid - qid po. **Muscle Spasms (Over 5 yrs):** 5 - 10 mg IM or slow IV. Repeat in 3 - 4 h, if necessary. **Tetanus in Infants Over 30 days old:** 1 - 2 mg IM or slow IV, repeated q 3 - 4 h prn. **Status Epilepticus and Severe Recurrent Convulsive Seizures:** **30 days - 5 yrs:** 0.2 - 0.5 mg by slow IV up to a maximum of 5 mg. Repeat in 2 - 4 h if necessary. **Over 5 yrs:** 1 mg by slow IV q 2 - 5 minutes up to a maximum of 10 mg. Repeat in 2 to 4 h if necessary.
	DIASTAT	Antiepileptic	**Rectal Gel (Pediatric):** 2.5, 5, 10 mg	**2-5 yrs:** Administer 0.5 mg/kg rectally. **6-11 yrs:** Administer 0.3 mg/kg rectally. Calculate the recommended dose by rounding up to the next available unit dose. A second dose, when required, may be given 4 - 12 h after the first dose. Do not treat more than 5 episodes/month or more than 1 episode q 5 days.
Diazoxide	HYPERSTAT i.V.	Antihypertensive	**Inj:** 300 mg/20 mL	1 - 3 mg/kg IV repeated at intervals of 5 - 15 min. Maximum: 150 mg in a single injection.
	PROGLYCEM	Hyperglycemic Agent	**Susp:** 50 mg/mL	Infants & Newborns: 8 - 15 mg/kg daily po in 2 or 3 equal doses q 8 - 12 h. Children: 3 - 8 mg/kg/day po in 2 or 3 equal doses q 8 - 12 h.

GENERIC NAME	COMMON TRADE NAMES	THERAPEUTIC CATEGORY	PREPARATIONS	COMMON PEDIATRIC DOSAGE
Dibucaine	NUPERCAINAL	Local Anesthetic (Topical)	Cream: 0.5%	Apply to affected areas prn and rub in gently. Not more than 1/6 tube should be applied in 24 h.
			Oint: 1%	**Over 2 yrs:** Apply to affected areas up to tid or qid.
Dicloxacillin Sodium	DYNAPEN, PATHOCIL	Antibacterial	Powd for Susp: 62.5 mg/5 mL Cpsl: 250, 500 mg	**Mild to Moderate Infections:** Under 40 kg: 12.5 mg/kg/day po in equally divided doses q 6 h. Over 40 kg: 125 mg q 6 h po. **More Severe Infections:** Under 40 kg: 25 mg/kg/day po in equally divided doses q 6 h. Over 40 kg: 250 mg q 6 h po.
Didanosine	VIDEX	Antiviral	Chewable / Dispersible Tab: 25, 50, 100, 150 mg	Based on body surface area and an oral dosage of 200 mg/m^2/day: < 0.4 m^2: 25 mg tabs bid. 0.5 - 0.7 m^2: 50 mg tabs bid. 0.8 - 1.0 m^2: 75 mg tabs bid. 1.1 - 1.4 m^2: 100 mg tabs bid. To prevent degradation by gastric acid, children under 1 year of age should take 1 tab and over 1 year old should take 2 tabs. Chew or crush and disperse 1 or 2 tabs in at least 1 fl. oz. of water prior to consumption. Take on an empty stomach.

| | | Pediatric Powd for Soln: 2, 4 g packets | Based on body surface area and an oral dosage of 200 mg/m²/day: |

Drug	Class	Forms	Dosage
Diflorasone Diacetate	Corticosteroid	Cream & Oint: 0.05% Emollient Cream: 0.05%	Apply to the affected area once daily to qid, depending on the severity of the condition. Apply to the affected area once daily to tid, depending on the severity of the condition.
Digoxin	Inotropic Agent	LANOXIN ELIXIR PEDIATRIC / LANOXIN — Elixir: 50 µg/mL (10% alcohol) Tab: 125, 250 µg Inj: 100, 250 µg/mL LANOXICAPS — Cpsl: 50, 100, 200 µg	**Doses by age:** see the Digoxin Table, p. 157. Recommended doses are average values that may require considerable modification because of individual sensitivity or associated conditions. **Under 10 yrs:** divided daily dosing is recommended. **Over 10 yrs:** generally once a day dosing is used.
Dimenhydrinate	Antivertigo Agent, Antiemetic	DRAMAMINE — Liquid: 12.5 mg/5 mL Chewable Tab & Tab: 50 mg Inj: 50 mg/mL	**2-6 yrs:** 12.5 - 25 mg q 6 - 8 h po. **6-12 yrs:** 25 - 50 mg q 6 - 8 h po. 1.25 mg/kg qid IM. Maximum: 300 mg.

Based on body surface area and an oral dosage of 200 mg/m²/day:

< 0.4 m²: 31 mg bid (in 3 mL mixture).
0.5 - 0.7 m²: 62 mg bid (in 6 mL mixture).
0.8 - 1.0 m²: 94 mg bid (in 9.5 mL mixture).
1.1 - 1.4 m²: 125 mg bid (in 12.5 mL mixture).

Dissolve contents of packet in water to make solution of 20 mg/mL; then mix with a liquid antacid to make a mixture of 10 mg/mL. Drink on an empty stomach.

GENERIC NAME	COMMON TRADE NAMES	THERAPEUTIC CATEGORY	PREPARATIONS	COMMON PEDIATRIC DOSAGE
Diphenhydramine Hydrochloride	BENADRYL ALLERGY	Antihistamine	Liquid: 12.5 mg/5 mL	**6-12 yrs:** 12.5 - 25 mg (5 - 10 mL) q 4 - 6 h po, not to exceed 60 mL in 24 h.
			Chewable Tab: 12.5 mg	**6-12 yrs:** 12.5 - 25 mg q 4 - 6 h po, not to exceed 150 mg in 24 h.
			Cpsl & Tab: 25 mg	**6-12 yrs:** 12.5 * - 25 mg q 4 - 6 h po, not to exceed 150 mg in 24 h. [* The Liquid is recommended for this dosage].
	BENADRYL DYE-FREE		Liquid: 12.5 mg/5 mL	**6-12 yrs:** 12.5 - 25 mg (5 - 10 mL) q 4 - 6 h po, not to exceed 60 mL in 24 h.
			Soft-Gel Cpsl: 25 mg	**6-12 yrs:** 12.5 * - 25 mg q 4 - 6 h po, not to exceed 150 mg in 24 h. [* The Liquid is recommended for this dosage].
	BENADRYL		Inj: 10, 50 mg/mL	5 mg/kg/24 h or 150 mg/m^2 IV or by deep IM injection divided into 4 doses. Maximum daily dosage is 300 mg.
	BENADRYL ITCH STOPPING GEL - Original Strength		Gel: 1%	**Over 6 yrs:** Apply to affected areas not more than tid to qid.
Disopyramide Phosphate	NORPACE	Antiarrhythmic	Cpsl: 100, 150 mg	**Under 1 yr:** 10 - 30 mg/kg/day po in divided doses q 6 h. **1-4 yrs:** 10 - 20 mg/kg/day po in divided doses q 6 h. **4-12 yrs:** 10 - 15 mg/kg/day po in divided doses q 6 h. **12-18 yrs:** 6 - 15 mg/kg/day po in divided doses q 6 h.

52

Divalproex Sodium	DEPAKOTE	Antiepileptic	Delayed-Rel. Tab: 125, 250, 500 mg Sprinkle Cpsl: 125 mg	**Over 10 yrs:** Initially, 10 - 15 mg/kg/day po; increase at 1 week intervals by 5 - 10 mg/kg/day (Maximum: 60 mg/kg/day). If total daily dosage exceeds 250 mg, it should be given in divided doses.
Docusate Sodium	COLACE	Stool Softener	Liquid (Drops): 50 mg/5 mL Syrup: 20 mg/5 mL Cpsl: 50, 100 mg	**Under 3 yrs:** 10 - 40 mg po. **3-6 yrs:** 20 - 60 mg po. **6-12 yrs:** 40 - 120 mg po.
	COLACE MICROENEMA		Rectal Solution: 200 mg/5 mL	**3-12 yrs:** Slowly insert half-length of the nozzle into the rectum. Squeeze out the entire contents of the tube.
	CORRECTOL STOOL SOFTENER		Soft-Gel: 100 mg	**2-12 yrs:** 100 mg once daily po.
	DIALOSE		Tab: 100 mg	**2-12 yrs:** 100 mg once daily po.
	EX-LAX STOOL SOFTENER		Cplt: 100 mg	**2-12 yrs:** 100 mg once daily po.
	PHILLIPS LIQUI-GELS		Liqui-Gel: 100 mg	**2-12 yrs:** 100 mg once daily po.
Dolasetron Mesylate	ANZEMET	Antiemetic	Tab: 50, 100 mg	**Prevention of Chemotherapy-Induced Nausea and Vomiting (2-16 yrs):** 1.8 mg/kg po within 1 h before chemotherapy, up to a maximum of 100 mg. **Prevention or Treatment of Postoperative Nausea and Vomiting (2-16 yrs):** 1.2 mg/kg po within 2 h before surgery, up to a maximum of 100 mg.

53

[Continued on the next page]

GENERIC NAME	COMMON TRADE NAMES	THERAPEUTIC CATEGORY	PREPARATIONS	COMMON PEDIATRIC DOSAGE
Dolasetron Mesylate [Continued]			Inj: 20 mg/mL	**Prevention of Chemotherapy-Induced Nausea and Vomiting (2-16 yrs)**: 1.8 mg/kg IV as a single dose about 30 min before chemotherapy, up to a maximum of 100 mg. **Prevention or Treatment of Postoperative Nausea and Vomiting (2-16 yrs)**: 0.35 mg/kg IV as a single dose about 15 min before the cessation of anesthesia or as soon as nausea or vomiting presents, up to a maximum of 12.5 mg.
Dornase Alfa Recombinant	PULMOZYME	Drug for Cystic Fibrosis Patients	Solution for Inhalation: 1.0 mg/mL (2.5 mL amp)	One 2.5 mL ampule inhaled once daily using a recommended nebulizer.
Doxacurium Chloride	NUROMAX	Neuromuscular Blocker	Inj: 1 mg/mL	**2-12 yrs**: Initially, 0.03 - 0.05 mg/kg IV (depending on duration of effect desired and other drugs given). Maintenance doses are required more frequently in children than in adults.
Doxycycline Calcium	VIBRAMYCIN	Antibacterial, Antimalarial	Syrup: 50 mg/5 mL	**Over 8 yrs and Up to 100 lbs**: 2 mg/lb po divided into 2 doses on the 1st day, followed by 1 mg/lb given as a single daily dose or divided into 2 doses. For more severe infections, up to 2 mg/lb may be used. **Over 100 lbs**: Use Adult dosage below - **Usual Dosage**: 100 mg q 12 h po for the first day, followed by a maintenance dose of 100 mg/day given as 50 mg q 12 h or 100 mg once daily. **Malaria Prophylaxis**: 2 mg/kg/day po up to the adult dose of 100 mg once daily po. Prophylaxis should begin 1 - 2 days before travel to the malarious area and should continue for 4 weeks after the traveler leaves the malarious area.

54

Doxycycline Hyclate	VIBRAMYCIN VIBRA-TAB	Antibacterial, Antimalarial	Cpsl: 50, 100 mg Tab: 100 mg	Same dosages as for VIBRAMYCIN Syrup.
	VIBRAMYCIN INTRAVENOUS	Antibacterial	Powd for Inj: 100 mg	**Over 8 yrs and** **Up to 100 lbs:** 2 mg/lb administered in 1 or 2 IV infusions on the first day, followed by 1 - 2 mg/lb given as 1 or 2 IV infusions depending on the severity of the infection. **Over 100 lbs:** Use Adult dosage below - Usual Dosage: 200 mg on the first day given in 1 or 2 IV infusions, then 100 to 200 mg a day, with 200 mg given in 1 or 2 infusions.
Doxycycline Monohydrate	VIBRAMYCIN	Antibacterial, Antimalarial	Powd for Susp: 25 mg/5 mL	Same dosages as for VIBRAMYCIN Syrup.
	MONODOX		Cpsl: 50, 100 mg	Same dosages as for VIBRAMYCIN Syrup.
Dronabinol (C-II)	MARINOL	Antiemetic	Cpsl: 2.5, 5, 10 mg	5 mg/m² po, 1 - 3 h prior to chemotherapy, then q 2 - 4 h after chemotherapy for a total of 4 - 6 doses/day.
Dyclonine Hydrochloride	SUCRETS	Local Anesthetic (Oral)	Lozenge (Children's Cherry): 1.2 mg	**Over 2 yrs:** Dissolve 1 slowly in the mouth. May repeat q 2 h prn.
			Lozenge (Wild Cherry & Vapor Lemon): 2 mg	**Over 2 yrs:** Dissolve 1 slowly in the mouth. May repeat q 2 h prn.
			Lozenge (Wintergreen & Vapor Black Cherry): 3 mg	**Over 2 yrs:** Dissolve 1 slowly in the mouth. May repeat q 2 h prn.
	CEPACOL MAXIMUM STRENGTH SORE THROAT SPRAY		Liquid (with pump sprayer): 0.1% (Cherry & Cool Menthol flavors)	**2-12 yrs:** Spray 2 - 3 times into throat and swallow. Repeat prn up to qid.
Econazole Nitrate	SPECTAZOLE	Antifungal	Cream: 1%	**Tinea Infections:** Apply topically to the affected areas once daily. **Cutaneous Candidiasis:** Apply topically to the affected areas bid.

GENERIC NAME	COMMON TRADE NAMES	THERAPEUTIC CATEGORY	PREPARATIONS	COMMON PEDIATRIC DOSAGE
Edrophonium Chloride	TENSILON, ENLON	Cholinomimetic	**Inj**: 10 mg/mL	**Diagnosis of Myasthenia:** **Infants:** Recommended dose is 0.5 mg. **Up to 75 lbs:** 1 mg IV; if no reaction occurs after 45 seconds, titrate dose up to 5 mg, given in increments of 1 mg q 30 - 45 seconds. May give IM (2 mg) as above except there is a delay of 2 - 10 minutes before a reaction occurs. **Over 75 lbs:** 2 mg IV; if no reaction occurs after 45 seconds, titrate dose up to 10 mg, given in increments of 1 mg q 30 - 45 seconds. May give IM (5 mg) as above except there is a delay of 2 - 10 minutes before a reaction occurs.
Emedastine Difumarate	EMADINE	Antihistamine	**Ophth Solution:** 0.05%	**Over 3 yrs:** 1 drop in the affected eye(s) up to qid.
Ephedrine Sulfate		Bronchodilator	**Cpsl:** 25, 50 mg **Inj:** 50 mg/mL	3 mg/kg/day in divided doses q 4 - 6 h po. 16.7 mg/m^2 in divided doses q 4 - 6 h SC or IV.
Epinephrine	SUS-PHRINE	Bronchodilator	**Inj:** 5 mg/mL (1:200)	**1 mo - 12 yrs:** 0.005 mL/kg SC. (For children under 30 kg, the maximum single dose is 0.15 mL).
	BRONKAID MIST PRIMATENE MIST	Bronchodilator	**Aerosol:** 0.25 mg/spray **Aerosol:** 0.22 mg/spray	**Over 4 yrs:** 1 inhalation, then wait at least 1 minute. If not relieved, use once more. Do not use again for at least 3 h.
Epinephrine Bitartrate	BRONKAID MIST SUSPENSION, PRIMATENE MIST SUSPENSION	Bronchodilator	**Aerosol:** 0.3 mg/spray (equal to 0.16 mg of epinephrine)	**Over 4 yrs:** 1 inhalation, then wait at least 1 minute. If not relieved, use once more. Do not use again for at least 3 h.

Epinephrine Hydrochloride	Sympathomimetic, Bronchodilator	EPIPEN, EPI E-Z PEN EPIPEN JR., EPI E-Z PEN JR.	**Auto-Injector:** 1:1000 soln (0.3 mg delivered per injection of 0.3 mL) **Auto-Injector:** 1:2000 soln (0.15 mg delivered per injection of 0.3 mL)	The appropriate dosage may be 0.15 or 0.30 mg depending on the body weight of the patient. However, the prescribing physician has the option of prescribing more or less than these amounts, based on a careful assessment of each patient.
		ADRENALIN CHLORIDE	**Solution:** 1:100 (10 mg/mL)	Variable by nebulizer.
			Inj: 1:1000 (1 mg/mL)	0.01 mg/kg SC (maximum: 0.5 mg); repeat q 20 min to 4 h prn.
Erythromycin	Antibacterial	ERY-TAB	**Delayed-Rel. Tab:** 250, 333, 500 mg	**Usual Dosage:** 30 - 50 mg/kg/day po in divided doses q 6 - 12 h for 10 - 14 days. **More Severe Infections:** The above dose may be doubled.
		ERYC	**Delayed-Rel. Cpsl:** 250 mg	Same dosages as for ERY-TAB above.
		ERYTHROMYCIN DELAYED-RELEASE	**Cpsl:** 250 mg	Same dosages as for ERY-TAB above.
		ERYTHROMYCIN BASE FILMTAB	**Tab:** 250, 500 mg	Same dosages as for ERY-TAB above given q 6 h po. If a bid schedule is desired, one-half the total daily dose may be given q 12 h po, 1 h ac.
		PCE	**Dispersable Tab:** 333, 500 mg	Same dosages as for ERY-TAB above.
		ILOTYCIN	**Ophth Oint:** 5 mg/g (0.5%)	**Neonates (Prophylaxis of Neonatal Gonococcal or Chlamydial Conjunctivitis):** Place a 1 - 2 cm ribbon of ointment into each lower conjunctival sac. Do not flush from the eye following instillation. **Older children:** Apply approx. 1 cm of ointment to the infected eye(s) up to 6 times daily, depending on the severity of the infection.

57

GENERIC NAME	COMMON TRADE NAMES	THERAPEUTIC CATEGORY	PREPARATIONS	COMMON PEDIATRIC DOSAGE
Erythromycin Estolate	ILOSONE	Antibacterial	Susp (per 5 mL): 125, 250 mg Cpsl: 250 mg Tab: 500 mg	**Usual Dosage:** 30 - 50 mg/kg/day po in divided doses q 6 - 12 h for 5 to 14 days, depending on the infection. If a bid schedule is desired, one-half the total daily dose may be given q 12 h po. **More Severe Infections:** The above dose may be doubled.
Erythromycin Ethylsuccinate	E.E.S.	Antibacterial	Powd for Susp: 200 mg Susp (per 5 mL): 200, 400 mg Tab: 400 mg	**Usual Dosage:** 30 - 50 mg/kg/day po in divided doses q 6 h for 5 - 14 days, depending on the infection. If a bid schedule is desired, one-half the total daily dose may be given q 12 h po. Doses may be given tid by giving one-third the total daily dose q 8 h. **Daily Dose by Weight:** Under 10 lbs: 15 - 25 mg/lb/day (30 - 50 mg/kg/day). 10 - 15 lbs: 200 mg. 16 - 25 lbs: 400 mg. 26 - 50 lbs: 800 mg. 51 - 100 lbs: 1200 mg. Over 100 lbs: 1600 mg. **More Severe Infections:** The above dose may be doubled.
	ERYPED		**Powd for Susp (Drops):** 100 mg/2.5 mL **Powd for Susp (per 5 mL):** 200, 400 mg **Chewable Tab:** 200 mg	Same dosages as for E.E.S. above.
Erythromycin Gluceptate	ILOTYCIN GLUCEPTATE	Antibacterial	Powd for Inj: 1 g	15 - 20 mg/kg/day by continuous IV infusion or in divided doses q 6 h IV.
Erythromycin Lactobionate		Antibacterial	Powd for Inj: 500 mg: 1 g	**Severe Infections:** 15-20 mg/kg/day by contin. IV infusion or by intermittent IV infusion in 20 - 60 min periods at intervals of ≤ 6 h.

58

Erythromycin Stearate	ERYTHROCIN STEARATE	Antibacterial	**Tab:** 250, 500 mg	**Mild to Moderate Infections:** 30 - 50 mg/kg/day po in 3 or 4 divided doses for 7 to 10 days depending on the infection. If a bid schedule is desired, one-half the total daily dose may be given q 12 h po on an empty stomach or immediately ac. **More Severe Infections:** The above dose may be doubled.
Ethacrynic Acid	EDECRIN	Diuretic	**Tab:** 25, 50 mg	**Except for Infants:** Initially, 25 mg po. Careful stepwise dosage increments of 25 mg should be made to achieve maintenance dosage.
Ethosuximide	ZARONTIN	Antiepileptic	**Syrup:** 250 mg/5 mL **Cpsl:** 250 mg	**Initial (3-6 yrs):** 250 mg/day po. **Initial (6-12 yrs):** 500 mg/day po. **Maintenance Doses:** Dosage must be individualized according to the patient's response. Dose may be increased by small increments (e.g., 250 mg q 4 - 7 days) until control is achieved. The optimal dose for most children is 20 mg/kg/day po.
Ethotoin	PEGANONE	Antiepileptic	**Tab:** 250, 500 mg	**Initial:** Dose should not exceed 750 mg daily po. Take after food. **Maintenance:** 500 - 1000 mg/day po in 4 - 6 equally divided doses after food.
Felbamate	FELBATROL	Antiepileptic	**Tab:** 400, 600 mg **Susp:** 600 mg/5 mL	**Adjunctive Therapy in Lennox-Gastaut Syndrome (2-14 yrs):** Add at 15 mg/kg/day po in divided doses tid or qid while reducing present antiepileptic drugs by 20% in order to control plasma levels of concurrent phenytoin, valproic acid, and carbamazepine. Increase the dosage of felbamate by 15 mg/kg/day increments at weekly intervals to 45 mg/kg/day.

GENERIC NAME	COMMON TRADE NAMES	THERAPEUTIC CATEGORY	PREPARATIONS	COMMON PEDIATRIC DOSAGE
Fentanyl Citrate (C-II)	SUBLIMAZE	Opioid Analgesic	**Inj**: 50 µg/mL (as the base)	**2-12 yrs**: Doses as low as 2 - 3 µg/kg IM or IV are recommended.
	FENTANYL ORALET	Opioid Analgesic	**Lozenge**: 100, 200, 300, 400 µg	**Over 15 kg**: Administer only in a hospital setting. Individualize dosage: usually 5 to 15 µg/kg po (sucking) 20 - 40 min prior to the anticipated need of desired effect. The premedication of children under 40 kg may require 10 - 15 µg/kg.
Ferrous Sulfate (20% iron)	FER-IN-SOL	Hematinic	**Liquid (Drops)**: 75 mg/0.6 mL **Syrup**: 90 mg/5 mL (5% alcohol)	**6 mos - 2 yrs**: Up to 6 mg/kg/day po in 3 - 4 divided doses. **2-12 yrs (15-30 kg)**: 3 mg/kg/day po in 3 - 4 divided doses.
	FEOSOL		**Elixir**: 220 mg/5 mL (5% alcohol)	**6 mos - 2 yrs**: Up to 6 mg/kg/day po in 3 - 4 divided doses. **2-12 yrs (15-30 kg)**: 3 mg/kg/day po in 3 - 4 divided doses.
Ferrous Sulfate, Exsiccated (30% iron)	FER-IN-SOL	Hematinic	**Cpsl**: 190 mg	**4-12 yrs**: 1 cpsl daily po.
	FEOSOL		**Tab**: 200 mg	**6-12 yrs**: 1 tab tid pc po.
	SLOW FE		**Slow Rel. Tab**: 160 mg	**6-12 yrs**: 1 tab daily po.
Fluconazole	DIFLUCAN	Antifungal	**Tab**: 50, 100, 150, 200 mg **Powd for Susp**: 10, 40 mg/mL **Inj**: 200 mg/100 mL, 400 mg/200 mL	**Oropharyngeal Candidiasis**: 6 mg/kg on the first day, followed by 3 mg/kg once daily po or IV. Continue treatment for at least 2 weeks. **Esophageal Candidiasis**: 6 mg/kg on the first day, followed by 3 mg/kg once daily po or IV. Doses up to 12 mg/kg/day may be used based on the patient response. Continue treatment for a minimum of 3 weeks and at least 2 weeks following resolution of symptoms.

60

			Systemic Candidiasis: 6 - 12 mg/kg/day po or IV.
			Cryptococcal Meningitis: 12 mg/kg on the first day, followed by 6 mg/kg once daily po or IV. Continue therapy for 10 - 12 weeks after the cerebrospinal fluid becomes culture negative.
Flunisolide	AEROBID	Corticosteroid	Aerosol: 250 μg/spray	6-15 yrs: 2 inhalations bid AM and PM.
	NASALIDE, NASAREL		Nasal Spray: 0.025% (25 μg/spray)	6-14 yrs: 1 spray in each nostril tid or 2 sprays in each nostril bid.
Fluocinolone Acetonide	SYNALAR	Corticosteroid	Cream: 0.01, 0.025%	Apply as a thin film bid - qid.
			Oint: 0.025%	Apply as a thin film bid - qid.
			Topical Solution: 0.01%	Apply as a thin film bid - qid.
	SYNALAR-HP		Cream: 0.2%	Over 2 yrs: Apply as a thin film bid - qid.
Fluocinonide	LIDEX	Corticosteroid	Cream, Oint, Gel & Solution: 0.05%	Apply as a thin film bid - qid.
Fluorometholone	FML	Corticosteroid	Ophth Oint: 0.1%	Over 2 yrs: Apply 1/2 inch ribbon to the eye(s) q 4 h for the 1st 24 - 48 h. When a favorable response is observed, reduce the dosage to 1 - 3 times daily.
			Ophth Susp: 0.1%	Over 2 yrs: 1 drop into the eye(s) bid - qid.
	FML FORTE		Ophth Susp: 0.25%	Over 2 yrs: 1 drop into the eye(s) bid - qid.
Flurandrenolide	CORDRAN	Corticosteroid	Cream & Oint: 0.025, 0.05% Lotion: 0.05%	Apply as a thin film to affected areas bid - tid and rub in gently.
			Tape: 4 mcg/cm²	Apply to affected areas; replace q 12 h.

GENERIC NAME	COMMON TRADE NAMES	THERAPEUTIC CATEGORY	PREPARATIONS	COMMON PEDIATRIC DOSAGE
Fluticasone Propionate	FLONASE	Corticosteroid	**Nasal Spray:** 0.05%	**Over 4 years:** 1 spray in each nostril once a day.
Fluvoxamine Maleate	LUVOX	Drug for Obsessive-Compulsive Disorder	**Tab:** 25, 50, 100 mg	**Over 8 yrs:** Initially, 25 mg hs po. Increase dose in 25 mg increments q 4 - 7 days, as tolerated, until maximum therapeutic benefit occurs. Daily dosages over 50 mg should be given in divided doses (bid). If the two divided doses are not equal, the larger dose should be given hs. Maximum: 200 mg/day.
Folic Acid		Vitamin	**Tab:** 0.4, 0.8, 1 mg	**Therapeutic Dosage:** Up to 1 mg daily po. **Maintenance Dosage:** **Under 4 yrs:** Up to 0.3 mg/day po. **Over 4 yrs:** 0.4 mg/day po.
Furazolidone	FUROXONE	Antibacterial	**Liquid:** 50 mg/15 mL	**1 mo - 1 yr:** 2.5 - 5 mL qid po. **1-4 yrs:** 5 - 7.5 mL qid po. **Over 4 yrs:** 7.5 - 15 mL qid po.
			Tab: 100 mg	**Over 4 yrs:** 25 - 50 mg qid po. (The above dosages are based on an average dose of 5 mg/kg given in 4 equally divided doses in 24 h).
Furosemide	LASIX	Diuretic	**Solution:** 10 mg/mL (11.5% alcohol) **Tab:** 20, 40, 80 mg	The usual initial dose is 2 mg/kg/day as a single po dose. Dosage may be increased by 1 or 2 mg/kg no sooner than 6 - 8 h after the previous dose. Maximum: 6 mg/kg.
			Inj: 10 mg/mL	The usual initial dose is 1 mg/kg by IM or slow IV injection. Dosage may be increased by 1 mg/kg no sooner than 2 h after the previous dose. Maximum: 6 mg/kg.

Gentamicin Sulfate	GARAMYCIN	Antibacterial	**Cream & Oint:** 0.1%	Apply to affected areas tid to qid.
	GARAMYCIN, GENTACIDIN		**Ophth Solution:** 3 mg/mL	1 - 2 drops into affected eye(s) q 4 h. In severe infections, dosage may be increased to as much as 2 drops once every hour.
			Ophth Oint: 3 mg/g	Apply to affected eye(s) bid or tid.
	GARAMYCIN I.V.		**Inj:** 40 mg/mL **Inj:** 10 mg/mL	**Neonates:** Birth - 7 days: 2.5 mg/kg q 12 h IM or IV. Over 7 days: 2.5 mg/kg q 8 h IM or IV. Older Neonates and Children: 2 - 2.5 mg/kg q 8 h IM or IV.
Glycerin	FLEET BABYLAX	Laxative	**Rectal Suppos:** (with sodium stearate)	Insert 1 suppository rectally prn.
			Rectal Liquid: (pure) in 4 mL rectal applicators	**2-6 yrs:** Insert tip rectally and administer the contents of one applicator (4 mL) in a single daily dose.
	FLEET GLYCERIN LAXATIVE RECTAL APPLICATORS		**Rectal Liquid:** (pure) in 7.6 mL rectal applicators	**6-12 yrs:** Insert tip rectally and administer the contents of one applicator (7.6 mL) in a single daily dose.
Gold Sodium Thiomalate		Antirheumatic	**Inj (per mL):** 25, 50 mg	After a test dose of 10 mg, give 1 mg/kg IM, not to exceed 50 mg for a single injection.
Granisetron Hydrochloride	KYTRIL	Antiemetic	**Inj:** 1.12 mg/mL (1 mg/mL as the base)	**2-16 yrs:** 10 μg/kg, infused IV over 5 minutes, beginning within 30 minutes before initiation of chemotherapy, and only on the days that chemotherapy is given.
Griseofulvin Microsize	FULVICIN U/F, GRISACTIN	Antifungal	**Tab:** 250, 500 mg	**Over 2 yrs:** 5 mg/lb/day po (as a single daily dose).
	GRIFULVIN V, GRIVATE		**Susp:** 125 mg/5 mL **Tab:** 250, 500 mg	**Over 2 yrs:** 5 mg/lb/day po (as a single daily dose).

63

GENERIC NAME	COMMON TRADE NAMES	THERAPEUTIC CATEGORY	PREPARATIONS	COMMON PEDIATRIC DOSAGE
Griseofulvin Ultramicrosize	FULVICIN P/G	Antifungal	**Tab:** 125, 165, 250, 330 mg	**Over 2 yrs:** 3.3 mg/lb/day po (as a single daily dose).
	GRIS-PEG		**Tab:** 125, 250 mg	**Over 2 yrs:** 3.3 mg/lb/day po (as a single daily dose). Dosage based on weight: 35-60 lbs: 125 - 187.5 mg daily po. > 60 lbs: 187.5 - 375 mg daily po.
	GRISACTIN ULTRA		**Tab:** 250, 330 mg	**Over 2 yrs:** 3.3 mg/lb/day po (as a single daily dose).
Guaifenesin	ROBITUSSIN	Expectorant	**Syrup:** 100 mg/5 mL	**2-6 yrs:** 2.5 - 5 mL q 4 h po. **6-12 yrs:** 5 - 10 mL q 4 h po.
	ORGANIDIN NR		**Liquid:** 100 mg/5 mL	**6 mos - 2 yrs:** 25 - 50 mg (1.25 - 2.5 mL) q 4 h po. **2-6 yrs:** 50 - 100 mg (2.5 - 5 mL) q 4 h po. **6-12 yr:** 100 - 200 mg (5 - 10 mL) q 4 h po.
	HUMIBID SPRINKLE		**Sustained-Rel. Cpsl:** 300 mg	**2-6 yrs:** 300 mg q 12 h po. **6-12 yrs:** 600 mg q 12 h po.
	HUMIBID L.A.		**Sustained-Rel. Tab:** 600 mg	**2-6 yrs:** 300 mg q 12 h po. **6-12 yrs:** 600 mg q 12 h po.
	DURATUSS-G		**Long-Acting Tab:** 1200 mg	**6-12 yrs:** 600 mg q 12 h po.
Halcinonide	HALOG	Corticosteroid	**Cream:** 0.025, 0.1% **Oint & Solution:** 0.1%	Apply to affected areas bid to tid.
Haloperidol	HALDOL	Antipsychotic	**Tab:** 0.5, 1, 2, 5, 10, 20 mg	**3-12 yrs (15 - 40 kg):** 0.05 - 0.15 mg/kg/day po in 2 or 3 divided doses.
Haloperidol Lactate	HALDOL	Antipsychotic	**Liquid Conc:** 2 mg/mL	**3-12 yrs (15 - 40 kg):** 0.05 - 0.15 mg/kg/day po in 2 or 3 divided doses.

Heparin Sodium	Anticoagulant	Inj: 1000 - 40,000 Units/mL	General Guidelines: **Initial Dose:** 50 Units/kg by IV drip. **Maintenance Dose:** 100 Units/kg by IV drip q 4 h or 20,000 Units/m²/24 h infused continuously.
Hexylresorcinol	Local Anesthetic (Oral)	Lozenge (Original Mint): 2.4 mg	**Over 2 yrs:** Dissolve 1 slowly in the mouth. May repeat q 2 h prn.
Homatropine Hydrobromide	Mydriatic - Cycloplegic	Ophth Solution: 2%	**Refraction:** Instill 1 - 2 drops in the eye(s). May be repeated in 5 - 10 min. if necessary. **Uveitis:** Instill 1 - 2 drops in the eye(s) q 3 - 4 h.
Hydrochlorothiazide	Diuretic, Antihypertensive	Tab: 25, 50, 100 mg	0.5 - 1 mg/lb/day (1 - 2 mg/kg/day) po in a single dose or in 2 divided doses q 12 h, not to exceed 37.5 mg/day in infants up to 2 yrs old or 100 mg/day in children 2 - 12 yrs of age. Infants under 6 mos of age may require 1.5 mg/lb/day po in 2 divided doses.
Hydrocortisone	Corticosteroid		
HYDROCORTONE		Tab: 10 mg	Initial dosage varies from 20 - 240 mg daily po depending on the disease being treated and the patient's response.
CORTEF		Tab: 5, 10, 20 mg	
CORTIZONE FOR KIDS CORTIZONE-5		Cream: 0.5% Cream & Oint: 0.5%	**Over 2 yrs:** Apply to affected area not more than tid to qid.
CORTIZONE-10		Cream & Oint: 1%	**Over 2 yrs:** Apply to affected area not more than tid to qid.
CORT-DOME		Cream: 0.5, 1%	**Over 2 yrs:** Apply as a thin film to affected areas bid - qid.
CORTAID		Cream, Oint & Stick: 0.5, 1%	**Over 2 yrs:** Apply to affected area not more than tid - qid.
ANUSOL-HC 2.5%		Cream: 2.5%	Apply as a thin film to affected areas bid - qid.
HYTONE		Cream, Oint & Lotion: 2.5%	Apply as a thin film to affected areas bid - qid.

GENERIC NAME	COMMON TRADE NAMES	THERAPEUTIC CATEGORY	PREPARATIONS	COMMON PEDIATRIC DOSAGE
Hydrocortisone Acetate	HYDROCORTONE ACETATE	Corticosteroid	Inj (per mL): 25, 50 mg [low solubility; provides a prolonged effect]	**Only for Intra-articular, Intralesional and Soft Tissue Injection:** Dose and frequency of injection are variable and must be individualized on the basis of the disease and the response of the patient. The initial dosage varies from 5 - 75 mg a day.
Hydrocortisone Butyrate	LOCOID	Corticosteroid	Cream, Oint & Solution: 0.1%	Apply as a thin film to affected areas bid to tid.
Hydrocortisone Sodium Phosphate	HYDROCORTONE PHOSPHATE	Corticosteroid	Inj: 50 mg/mL [water soluble; rapid onset, short duration]	**For IV, IM & SC Injection:** Dose requirements are variable and must be individualized on the basis of the disease and the response of the patient. The initial dosage varies from 15 - 240 mg a day.
Hydrocortisone Sodium Succinate	SOLU-CORTEF	Corticosteroid	Powd for Inj: 100, 250, 500, 1000 mg [water soluble; rapid onset, short duration]	100 - 500 mg IM, IV, or by IV infusion. Repeat at intervals of 2, 4, or 6 h.
Hydrocortisone Valerate	WESTCORT	Corticosteroid	Cream & Oint: 0.2%	Apply as a thin film to affected areas bid to tid.
Hydroxyzine Hydrochloride	ATARAX	Sedative, Antipruritic, Antianxiety Agent	Syrup: 10 mg/5 mL (0.5% alcohol) Tab: 10, 25, 50, 100 mg	**Sedation:** 0.6 mg/kg po. **Anxiety and Pruritis:** Under 6 yrs: 50 mg/day po in divided doses. Over 6 yrs: 50 - 100 mg/day po in divided doses.
	VISTARIL	Sedative, Antiemetic, Antianxiety Agent	Inj (per mL): 25, 50 mg	**Sedation:** 0.6 mg/kg IM. **Nausea & Vomiting:** 0.5 mg/lb IM. **Anxiety (Pre- and Postoperative):** 0.5 mg/lb IM.

66

Drug	Brand	Class	Formulations	Dosing
Hydroxyzine Pamoate	VISTARIL	Sedative, Antipruritic, Antianxiety Agent	Susp: 25 mg/5 mL Cpsl: 25, 50, 100 mg	Sedation: 0.6 mg/kg po. Anxiety and Pruritis: Under 6 yrs: 50 mg/day po in divided doses. Over 6 yrs: 50 - 100 mg/day po in divided doses.
Hyoscyamine Sulfate	LEVSIN	Anticholinergic, Antispasmodic	Solution (Drops): 0.125 mg/mL (5% alcohol)	Under 2 yrs: 2.3 kg (5 lbs): 3 drops q 4 h po. 3.4 kg (7.5 lbs): 4 drops q 4 h po. 5 kg (11 lbs): 5 drops q 4 h po. 7 kg (15 lbs): 6 drops q 4 h po. 10 kg (22 lbs): 8 drops q 4 h po. 15 kg (33 lbs): 11 drops q 4 h po. 2-12 yrs: 0.25 - 1 mL q 4 h po.
			Elixir: 0.125 mg/5 mL (20% alcohol)	2-12 yrs: 1.25 - 5 mL q 4 h po or 1.25 mL/10 kg q 4 h po.
			Tab & Sublingual Tab: 0.125 mg	2-12 yrs: 1/2 - 1 tablet q 4 h po.
			Inj: 0.5 mg/mL	Preanesthetic: 5 µg/kg IV, 30 - 60 min prior to anesthesia.
	LEVSINEX TIMECAPS		Timed-Rel. Cpsl: 0.375 mg	2-12 yrs: 1 capsule q 12 h po.
Ibuprofen	PEDIACARE FEVER DROPS	Antipyretic, Analgesic	Liquid (Drops): 50 mg/1.25 mL	2-3 yrs (24-35 lbs): 2.50 mL q 6 - 8 h po.
	CHILDREN'S MOTRIN		Liquid (Drops): 50 mg/1.25 mL	2-3 yrs (24-35 lbs): 2.50 mL q 6 - 8 h po.
			Susp: 100 mg/5 mL	2-3 yrs (24-35 lbs): 5 mL q 6 - 8 h po. 4-5 yrs (36-47 lbs): 7.5 mL q 6 - 8 h po. 6-8 yrs (48-59 lbs): 10 mL q 6 - 8 h po. 9-10 yrs (60-71 lbs): 12.5 mL q 6 - 8 h po. 11 yrs (72-95 lbs): 15 mL q 6 - 8 h po.

[Continued on the next page]

GENERIC NAME	COMMON TRADE NAMES	THERAPEUTIC CATEGORY	PREPARATIONS	COMMON PEDIATRIC DOSAGE
Ibuprofen [Continued]			Chewable Tab: 50 mg	4-5 yrs (36-47 lbs): 3 tabs q 6 - 8 h po. 6-8 yrs (48-59 lbs): 4 tabs q 6 - 8 h po. 9-10 yrs (60-71 lbs): 5 tabs q 6 - 8 h po. 11 yrs (72-95 lbs): 6 tabs q 6 - 8 h po.
	JUNIOR STRENGTH MOTRIN		Chewable Cplt & Tab: 100 mg	6-8 yrs (48-59 lbs): 2 cplts or tabs q 6 - 8 h po. 9-10 yrs (60-71 lbs): 2.5 cplts or tabs q 6 - 8 h po. 11 yrs (72-95 lbs): 3 cplts or tabs q 6 - 8 h po.
	CHILDREN'S ADVIL		Susp: 100 mg/5 mL	Same dosages as for CHILDREN'S MOTRIN above.
			Chewable Tab: 100 mg	6-10 yrs (48-71 lbs): 2 tabs q 6 - 8 h po. 11 yrs (72-95 lbs): 3 tabs q 6 - 8 h po.
	MOTRIN	Antipyretic, Analgesic, Nonsteroidal Anti-Inflammatory Drug	Oral Drops: 40 mg/mL Susp: 100 mg/5 mL Chewable Tab: 50, 100 mg Cplt: 100 mg	Fever (6 mos - 12 yrs): 5 mg/kg po if the baseline body temperature is below 102.5 °F or or 10 mg/kg if the baseline body temp. is 102.5 °F or greater. The duration of fever reduction is generally 6 - 8 h. The maximum daily dose is 40 mg/kg po. Mild to Moderate Pain (6 mos - 12 yrs): 10 mg/kg q 6 - 8 h po. The maximum daily dose is 40 mg/kg po. Juvenile Arthritis: 30 - 40 mg/kg/day divided into 3 or 4 doses po. Patients with mild disease may be treated with 20 mg/kg/day.
Imipramine Hydrochloride	TOFRANIL	Anti-Enuretic Agent	Tab: 10, 25, 50 mg	6-12 yrs: Initially 25 mg po one hour before bedtime. Dose may be increased to 50 mg po after 1 week, if necessary.
Insulin	ILETIN, HUMULIN, etc.	Hypoglycemic	Inj: 100 Units/mL	Variable; See the Insulin Table, pp. XXX - YYY for preparations.

Iodoquinol	YODOXIN	Amebicide	**Tab:** 210 mg	**Under 6 yrs:** 210 mg/15 lbs tid po after meals for 20 days. **6-12 yrs:** 420 mg tid po after meals for 20 days.
			Tab: 650 mg	40 mg/kg/day po divided into 3 doses (not to exceed 1.95 g per 24 h) taken after meals for 20 days.
Ipecac		Emetic	**Syrup:** approximately 40 mg of alkaloids/30 mL	**6 mos - 1 yr:** 10 mL po. **1-12 yrs:** 15 mL po. (Follow above doses with 100 to 150 mL of water; may repeat once in 20 minutes).
Isoniazid	INH	Tuberculostatic	**Tab:** 100, 300 mg	10 - 20 mg/kg (up to 300 mg) daily po.
	NYDRAZID		**Inj:** 100 mg/mL	**Treatment:** 10 - 20 mg/kg (up to 300 - 500 mg daily) depending on the severity of the infection IM in a single dose. **Preventive Therapy:** 10 mg/kg (up to 300 mg daily) IM in a single dose.
Isoproterenol Hydrochloride	ISUPREL	Bronchodilator	**Solution:** 1:200 (0.5%), 1:100 (1.0%)	**Acute Bronchial Asthma (Hand-Bulb Nebulizer):** 5 - 15 inhalations (of 1:200) up to 5 times daily. **Bronchospasm in COPD:** **Hand-Bulb Nebulizer: Same** dosage as for Acute Bronchial Asthma above. **Nebulization by Compressed Air or Oxygen:** 0.25 mL (of 1:200) diluted to 2 - 2.5 mL with water or isotonic saline. Flow rate is regulated to deliver over 10 - 15 minutes. Breath in mist up to 5 times daily. **IPPB:** 0.25 mL (of 1:200) diluted to 2 - 2.5 mL with water or isotonic saline. The IPPB treatments are usually given for 10 - 15 minutes, up to 5 times daily.
	ISUPREL MISTOMETER		**Aerosol:** 131 μg/spray	1 - 2 inhalations up to 5 times daily.

69

GENERIC NAME	COMMON TRADE NAMES	THERAPEUTIC CATEGORY	PREPARATIONS	COMMON PEDIATRIC DOSAGE
Ivermectin	STROMECTOL	Anthelmintic	Tab: 6 mg	Take po as a single daily dose with water; see the Table below.

Dosage for Strongyloidiasis

Body Weight (kg)	Number of Tablets
15 to 24	0.5
25 to 35	1
36 to 50	1.5
51 to 65	2
66 to 79	2.5
≥ 80	[200 μg/kg]

Dosage for Onchocerciasis

Body Weight (kg)	Number of Tablets
15 to 25	0.5
26 to 44	1
45 to 64	1.5
65 to 84	2
≥ 85	[150 μg/kg]

GENERIC NAME	COMMON TRADE NAMES	THERAPEUTIC CATEGORY	PREPARATIONS	COMMON PEDIATRIC DOSAGE
Kanamycin Sulfate	KANTREX PEDIATRIC KANTREX	Antibacterial	Inj: 75 mg/2 mL. Powd for Inj: 500, 1000 mg	7.5 mg/kg q 12 h deep IM or slow IV (over 30 - 60 minutes).
Ketoconazole	NIZORAL	Antifungal	Tab: 200 mg	**Over 2 yrs:** 3.3 - 6.6 mg/kg daily po.
Lamivudine	EPIVIR	Antiviral	Solution: 10 mg/mL. Tab: 150 mg	**Over 3 mos:** 4 mg/kg (maximum of 150 mg) bid po with zidovudine.
Levothyroxine Sodium	LEVOTHROID, LEVOXYL	Thyroid Hormone	Tab: 25, 50, 75, 88, 100, 112, 125, 137, 150, 175, 200, 300 μg	**Congenital Hypothyroidism:** **Birth - 6 mos:** 8 - 10 μg/kg/day po (25 - 50 μg per day po). **6-12 mos:** 6 - 8 μg/kg/day po (50 - 75 μg per day po). **1-5 yrs:** 5 - 6 μg/kg/day po (75 - 100 μg per day po). **6-12 yrs:** 4 - 5 μg/kg/day po (100 - 150 μg per day po).
	SYNTHROID		Tab: 25, 50, 75, 88, 100, 112, 125, 150, 175, 200, 300 μg	**Cretinism or Severe Hypothyroidism:** Initially 25 - 50 μg po with increases of 50 - 100 μg at weekly intervals until the patient is euthyroid. In growing children, the usual maintenance dose may be as high as 300 to 400 μg daily.

Lidocaine	XYLOCAINE	Local Anesthetic (Topical)	Oint: 2.5%	Apply topically prn.
			Oint: 5%	Apply topically. Maximum single application-determine by using Clark's rule, e.g., in a child of 5 yrs weighing 50 lbs, the maximum dose should not exceed 75 - 100 mg. In any case, the maximum amount should not exceed 4.5 mg/kg (2.0 mg/lb).
Lidocaine Hydrochloride	XYLOCAINE	Antiarrhythmic	Inj: 10, 20 mg	Bolus of 1.0 mg/kg IV followed by an IV infusion rate of 30 μg/kg/min.
	4% XYLOCAINE-MPF	Local Anesthetic (Injectable)	Inj: 40 mg/mL (4%)	Maximum recommended dosage is determined by using Clark's rule, e.g., in a child of 5 yrs weighing 50 lbs, the maximum dose should not exceed 75 - 100 mg. In any case, the maximum dose with epinephrine should not exceed 7 mg/kg (3.2 mg/lb); the maximum dose without epinephrine should not exceed 4.5 mg/kg (2.0 mg/lb).
	XYLOCAINE 2% VISCOUS	Local Anesthetic (Topical)	Solution: 2%	**Over 3 yrs:** Maximum recommended dosage-determine by using Clark's rule, e.g., in a child of 5 yrs weighing 50 lbs, the maximum dose should not exceed 75 - 100 mg (3.75 to 5 mL). **Under 3 yrs:** Apply 1.25 mL (accurately measured) to the area with a cotton-tipped applicator. May repeat dose no sooner than q 3 h.

GENERIC NAME	COMMON TRADE NAMES	THERAPEUTIC CATEGORY	PREPARATIONS	COMMON PEDIATRIC DOSAGE
Lincomycin Hydrochloride	LINCOCIN	Antibacterial	Cpsl: 500 mg	**Serious Infections (Over 1 mo):** 30 mg/kg/day po divided into 3 or 4 equal doses. **More Severe Infections (Over 1 mo):** 60 mg/kg/day po divided into 3 or 4 doses.
			Inj: 300 mg/mL	**Serious Infections (Over 1 mo):** 10 mg/kg IM q 24 h; or, 10 - 20 mg/kg per day by IV infusion (at a rate of 1 g/100 mL/hour). **More Severe Infections (Over 1 mo):** 10 mg/kg IM q 12 h or more often; or, 10 - 20 mg/kg per day by IV infusion (at a rate of 1 g/100 mL/hour).
Lindane		Antiparasitic, Scabicide	Lotion: 1%	**Scabies:** Apply to dry skin as a thin layer and rub in thoroughly. Leave on for 8 - 12 h, then remove by thorough washing.
			Shampoo: 1%	**Head & Crab Lice:** Apply 30 - 60 mL to dry hair. Work thoroughly into hair and allow to remain in place for 4 minutes. Add small amounts of water to form a good lather. Rinse thoroughly and towel dry.
Liothyronine Sodium	CYTOMEL	Thyroid Hormone	Tab: 5, 25, 50 μg	**Congenital Hypothyroidism:** 5 μg daily po and increase by 5 μg q 3 - 4 days until the desired response is obtained. Infants a few months old may need only 20 μg daily for maintenance; at 1 year, 50 μg daily may be required. Over 3 years, full adult dosage may be necessary.
Lodoxamide Tromethamine	ALOMIDE	Antiallergic	Ophth Solution: 0.1%	**Over 2 yrs:** 1 - 2 drops in each affected eye qid for up to 3 months.
Lomustine	CeeNU	Antineoplastic	Cpsl: 10, 40, 100 mg	130 mg/m² po as a single dose q 6 weeks. Dosage adjustments are made in 6 weeks based on platelet and leukocyte counts.

72

Loperamide Hydrochloride	IMODIUM A-D	Antidiarrheal	**Liquid:** 1 mg/5 mL (5.25% alcohol) **Cplt:** 2 mg	**2-5 yrs (24-47 lbs):** 1 mg (5 mL) po. Maximum: 3 mg (15 mL) daily. **6-8 yrs (48-59 lbs):** 2 mg (10 mL or 1 cplt or cpsl po. Maximum: 20 mL or 2 cplts or or cpsls daily.
	IMODIUM		**Cpsl:** 2 mg	**9-11 yrs (60-95 lbs):** 2 mg (10 mL or 1 cplt or cpsl po. Maximum: 30 mL or 3 cplts or cpsls daily.
	PEPTO DIARRHEA CONTROL		**Solution:** 1 mg/5 mL (5.25% alcohol) **Cplt:** 2 mg	The above doses should be given after each loose bowel movement up to the maximum per day.
	KAOPECTATE 1-D		**Cplt:** 2 mg	
Loracarbef	LORABID	Antibacterial	**Powd for Susp (per 5 mL):** 100, 200 mg **Cpsl:** 200, 400 mg	**Acute Otitis Media (6 mos - 12 yrs):** 30 mg/kg/day po (of the Suspension) in divided doses q 12 h for 10 days. **Pharyngitis & Tonsillitis (6 mos - 12 yrs):** 15 mg/kg/day po in divided doses q 12 h for 10 days. **Impetigo (6 mos - 12 yrs):** 15 mg/kg/day po in divided doses q 12 h for 7 days.
Loratadine	CLARITIN	Antihistamine	**Syrup:** 1 mg/mL **Tab:** 10 mg	**6-11 yrs:** 10 mL (10 mg) once daily po. **12 yrs:** 10 mg once daily po.
Lypressin	DIAPID	Posterior Pituitary Hormone	**Nasal Spray:** 0.185 mg/mL	**Over 6 wks:** 1 - 2 sprays in one or both nostrils qid. An additional dose hs often eliminates nocturia.
Mafenide Acetate	SULFAMYLON	Burn Preparation	**Cream:** 85 mg/g	Apply to the clean and debrided wound with a sterile gloved hand, once or twice daily, to a thickness of about 1/16 in.
Magnesium Hydroxide	MILK OF MAGNESIA	Saline Laxative	**Susp:** 400 mg/5 mL	**2-5 yrs:** 5 - 15 mL po. **6-11 yrs:** 15 - 30 mL po. **Over 11 yrs:** 30 - 60 mL po. (Follow the above doses with 8 oz. of liquid).
Magnesium Sulfate		Anticonvulsant	**Inj:** 1 mEq/mL (12.5%), 4 mEq/mL (50%)	20 - 40 mg/kg in a 20% solution IM; repeat prn.

73

GENERIC NAME	COMMON TRADE NAMES	THERAPEUTIC CATEGORY	PREPARATIONS	COMMON PEDIATRIC DOSAGE
Mebendazole	VERMOX	Anthelmintic	Chewable Tab: 100 mg	**Pinworm (Over 2 yrs):** 100 mg daily po (1 dose). **Common Roundworm, Whipworm, Hookworm (Over 2 yrs):** 100 mg bid AM and PM for 3 consecutive days po.
Mefloquine Hydrochloride	LARIAM	Antimalarial	Tab: 250 mg	**Prophylaxis:** Start with the following doses 1 week before travel and continue weekly during travel and for 4 weeks after leaving the area: 15 - 19 kg: 1/4 tablet po. 20 - 30 kg: 1/2 tablet po. 31 - 45 kg: 3/4 tablet po. > 45 kg: 1 tablet po.
Menthol	CEPACOL SORE THROAT LOZENGES (Regular Strength)	Local Anesthetic (Oral)	Lozenge (Original Mint): 2 mg	**Over 6 yrs:** Dissolve 1 in the mouth q 2 h prn.
			Lozenge (Cherry): 3.6 mg	**Over 6 yrs:** Dissolve 1 in the mouth q 2 h prn.
	HALLS JUNIORS	Antitussive	Lozenge: 2.5 mg	**Over 5 yrs:** Dissolve 2 (one at a time) slowly in the mouth. Repeat every hour prn.
	N'ICE	Local Anesthetic (Oral), Antitussive	Lozenge: 5 mg	**Sore Throat (Over 6 yrs):** Dissolve 1 slowly in the mouth. May repeat q 2 h, for up to 10 lozenges per day. **Cough (Over 6 yrs):** Dissolve 1 slowly in the mouth. May repeat every hour, for up to 10 lozenges per day.
	HALLS MENTHO-LYPTUS	Antitussive	Lozenge (Regular): 7 mg	**Over 5 yrs:** Dissolve 1 slowly in the mouth. Repeat every hour prn.
			Lozenge (Spearmint): 6 mg	**Over 5 yrs:** Dissolve 1 slowly in the mouth. Repeat every hour prn.
			Lozenge (Cherry): 7.6 mg	**Over 5 yrs:** Dissolve 1 slowly in the mouth. Repeat every hour prn.

		Lozenge (Honey-Lemon): 8.6 mg	**Over 5 yrs:** Dissolve 1 slowly in the mouth. Repeat every hour prn.
		Lozenge (Ice Blue Peppermint): 12 mg	**Over 5 yrs:** Dissolve 1 slowly in the mouth. Repeat every hour prn.
HALLS SUGAR FREE MENTHO-LYPTUS	Antitussive	**Lozenge (Black Cherry & Citrus Blend):** 5 mg	**Over 5 yrs:** Dissolve 1 slowly in the mouth. Repeat every hour prn.
		Lozenge (Mountain Menthol): 6 mg	**Over 5 yrs:** Dissolve 1 slowly in the mouth. Repeat every hour prn.
ROBITUSSIN COUGH DROPS	Antitussive	**Lozenge (Cherry & Menthol Eucalyptus):** 7.4 mg	**Over 4 yrs:** Dissolve 1 slowly in the mouth. May repeat every hour prn.
		Lozenge (Honey-Lemon): 10 mg	**Over 4 yrs:** Dissolve 1 slowly in the mouth. May repeat every hour prn.
ABSORBINE JR.	Local Anesthetic (Topical)	**Liquid:** 1.27%	**Over 2 yrs:** Apply to and gently massage the affected areas. Repeat prn up to qid.
DEMEROL Meperidine Hydrochloride (C-II)	Opioid Analgesic	**Tab:** 50, 100 mg **Syrup:** 50 mg/5 mL **Inj (per mL):** 25, 50, 75,	**Analgesia:** 0.5 - 0.8 mg/lb q 3 - 4 h po, SC or IM up to the adult dose of 50 - 100 mg. **Preoperatively:** 0.5 - 1.0 mg/lb IM or SC up to the adult dose of 50 - 100 mg. 30 - 90 minutes prior to anesthesia.
MESANTOIN Mephenytoin	Antiepileptic	**Tab:** 100 mg	Initially, 50 - 100 mg daily po, increasing the daily dose by 50 - 100 mg at weekly intervals to a maintenance dosage of 100 to 400 mg daily po.
MEBARAL Mephobarbital (C-IV)	Sedative, Antiepileptic	**Tab:** 32, 50, 100 mg	**Sedation:** 16 - 32 mg tid or qid po. **Epilepsy:** **Under 5 yrs:** 16 - 32 mg tid or qid po. **Over 5 yrs:** 32 - 64 mg tid or qid po.
EQUANIL, MILTOWN	Antianxiety Agent	**Tab:** 200, 400 mg	**Over 6 yrs:** 200 - 600 mg po in 2 or 3 divided doses.

GENERIC NAME	COMMON TRADE NAMES	THERAPEUTIC CATEGORY	PREPARATIONS	COMMON PEDIATRIC DOSAGE
Mercaptopurine	PURINETHOL	Antineoplastic	Tab: 50 mg	**Induction:** 2.5 mg/kg daily po. May increase after 4 weeks to 5 mg/kg daily po. **Maintenance:** 1.5 - 2.5 mg/kg po as a single dose.
Meropenem	MERREM IV	Antibacterial	Powd for Inj: 0.5, 1 g	**Intra-Abdominal Infection:** Over 3 mos: 20 mg/kg (Max: 2 g) q 8 h. Over 50 kg: 1 g q 8 h. **Meningitis:** Over 3 mos: 40 mg/kg (Max: 2 g) q 8 h. Over 50 kg: 2 g q 8 h. Give the above by IV infusion (over 15 - 30 min) or as an IV bolus (over 3 - 5 min).
Metaproterenol Sulfate	ALUPENT	Bronchodilator	Syrup: 10 mg/5 mL Tab: 10, 20 mg	**Under 6 yrs:** 1.3 - 2.6 mg/kg/day in divided doses po (Syrup only). **6-9 yrs (Under 60 lbs):** 10 mg tid or qid po. **Over 9 yrs (Over 60 lbs):** 20 mg tid or qid po.
Methamphetamine Hydrochloride (C-II)	DESOXYN	CNS Stimulant	Sustained-Rel. Tab: 5, 10, 15 mg	**Attention Deficit Disorder (Over 6 yrs):** Initially 5 mg once a day or twice a day po; the daily dose may be raised in increments of 5 mg at weekly intervals until the optimal clinical response is obtained. The usual effective dose is 20 - 25 mg daily.
Methenamine Hippurate	HIPREX, UREX	Urinary Anti-infective	Tab: 1 g	**6-12 yrs:** 0.5 - 1 g bid po.
Methenamine Mandelate	MANDELAMINE	Urinary Anti-infective	Susp: 500 mg/5 mL Tab: 0.5, 1 g	**Under 6 yrs:** 250 mg/30 lb qid po. **6-12 yrs:** 500 mg qid po.
Methimazole	TAPAZOLE	Antithyroid Agent	Tab: 5, 10 mg	**Initial Dose:** 0.4 mg/kg/day in divided doses q 8 h po. **Maintenance Dose:** Approximately 1/2 of the initial dose po.
Methionine	PEDAMETH	Diaper Rash Product	Liquid: 75 mg/5 mL	75 mg in liquids tid to qid po.

76

Methocarbamol	ROBAXIN INJECTABLE	Skeletal Muscle Relaxant	Inj: 100 mg/mL	A minimum initial dose of 15 mg/kg IV is recommended. May be repeated q 6 h.
Methsuximide	CELONTIN	Antiepileptic	Cpsl: 150, 300 mg	300 mg daily po for the 1st week. May raise dosage at weekly intervals by 300 mg/day for 3 weeks to a daily dosage of 1200 mg.
Methylcellulose	CITRUCEL	Bulk Laxative	Powder: 2 g/heaping tablespoonful (19 g)	6-12 yrs: 1/2 heaping tablespoonful stirred into 4 fl. oz. of cold water 1 - 3 times daily po.
	CITRUCEL (Sugar-Free)		Powder: 2 g/heaping tablespoonful (10.2 g)	6-12 yrs: 1/2 heaping tablespoonful stirred into 4 fl. oz. of cold water 1 - 3 times daily po.
Methyldopa	ALDOMET	Antihypertensive	Susp: 250 mg/5 mL (1% alcohol) Tab: 125, 250, 500 mg	Initial dose is 10 mg/kg/day po in 2 to 4 divided doses. Maximum dosage is 65 mg/kg or 3 g daily, whichever is less.
Methyldopate Hydrochloride	ALDOMET	Antihypertensive	Inj: 250 mg/5 mL	20 - 40 mg/kg/day in divided doses q 6 h IV in D_5W given over 30 - 60 minutes. Maximum dosage is 65 mg/kg or 3 g daily, whichever is less.
Methylphenidate Hydrochloride (C-II)	RITALIN	CNS Stimulant	Tab: 5, 10, 20 mg	**Attention Deficit Disorder (Over 6 yrs):** 5 mg bid po; may increase the daily dose by 5 mg weekly, not to exceed 60 mg per day.
	RITALIN-SR		Sustained-Rel. Tab: 20 mg	Since the duration of action of this preparation is approximately 8 h, it may be used in place of RITALIN tablets when the 8-hour dosage of RITALIN SR corresponds to the titrated 8-hour dosage of RITALIN.
Methylprednisolone	MEDROL	Corticosteroid	Tab: 2, 4, 8, 16, 24, 32 mg	Initial dosage varies from 4 - 48 mg daily po, depending on the disease being treated. This dosage should be maintained or adjusted until the patient's response is satisfactory.

77

GENERIC NAME	COMMON TRADE NAMES	THERAPEUTIC CATEGORY	PREPARATIONS	COMMON PEDIATRIC DOSAGE
Methylprednisolone Acetate	DEPO-MEDROL	Corticosteroid	Inj (per mL): 20, 40, 80 mg [low solubility; provides a prolonged effect]	**Only for Intra-articular, Intralesional and Soft Tissue Injection:** Dose and frequency of injection are variable and must be individualized on the basis of the disease and the response of the patient.
Methylprednisolone Sodium Succinate	SOLU-MEDROL	Corticosteroid	Powd for Inj: 40, 125, 500 mg; 1, 2 g [water soluble: rapid effect]	**For IV or IM Use:** The usual dose is 30 mg/kg IV (administered over at least 30 minutes) q 4 - 6 h for 48 hours. The dosage may be reduced for infants and children but the minimum dose is 0.5 mg/kg/24 hours in divided doses IM or IV; dosage is governed by the severity of the condition and the response of the patient.
Metoclopramide Hydrochloride	REGLAN	Gastrointestinal Stimulant	Inj: 5 mg/mL	**To Facilitate Small Bowel Intubation:** 1-6 yrs: 0.1 mg/kg by slow IV injection. 6-14 yrs: 2.5 - 5 mg by slow IV injection.
Metocurine Iodide	METUBINE IODIDE	Neuromuscular Blocker	Inj: 2 mg/mL	0.2 - 0.4 mg/kg IV (over 30 - 60 seconds). Supplemental doses (average, 0.5 - 1 mg) may be made as required.
Metronidazole	FLAGYL	Amebicide	Tab: 250, 500 mg	35 - 50 mg/kg/day in 3 divided doses (q 8 h) po for 10 days.
Mezlocillin Sodium	MEZLIN	Antibacterial	Powd for Inj: 1, 2, 3, 4 g	Neonates (Birth - 7 days): 75 mg/kg q 12 h IM or IV. Neonates (Over 7 days) and Under 2 kg: 75 mg/kg q 8 h IM or IV. Over 2 kg: 75 mg/kg q 6 h IM or IV. Over 1 mo: 50 mg/kg q 4 h IM or IV.
Miconazole	MONISTAT I.V.	Antifungal	Inj: 10 mg/mL	Under 1 yr: 15 - 30 mg/kg/day in divided doses q 8 h by IV infusion have been used. Over 1 yr: 20 - 40 mg/kg/day in divided doses q 8 h by IV infusion.

Miconazole Nitrate	MONISTAT-DERM	Antifungal	**Cream:** 2%	**Over 2 yrs:** Apply to affected areas bid, AM and PM.
	DESENEX, LOTRIMIN AF		**Spray Powd & Spray Liq:** 2%	**Over 2 yrs:** Spray a thin layer over affected area bid, AM and PM.
	CRUEX		**Spray Powd:** 2%	**Over 2 yrs:** Spray a thin layer over affected area bid, AM and PM.
	MICATIN		**Cream, Powder & Spray:** 2%	**Over 2 yrs:** Apply to affected areas bid, AM and PM.
Mineral Oil	FLEET MINERAL OIL ENEMA	Emollient Laxative	**Rectal Liquid:** (pure)	2-12 yrs: Administer 1/2 bottle (59 mL) rectally as a single dose.
Minocycline Hydrochloride	MINOCIN	Antibacterial	**Susp:** 50 mg/5 mL (5% alcohol) **Cpsl:** 50, 100 mg **Powd for Inj:** 100 mg	**Over 8 yrs:** Usually 4 mg/kg initially; then 2 mg/kg q 12 h po or IV.
Minoxidil	LONITEN	Antihypertensive	**Tab:** 2.5, 10 mg	The initial dosage is 0.2 mg/kg po as a single daily dose. The dosage may be increased in 50 - 100% increments until optimum blood pressure control is achieved. The effective dosage range is usually 0.25 - 1.0 mg/kg daily po (Maximum: 50 mg/day).
Mivacurium Chloride	MIVACRON	Neuromuscular Blocker	**Inj:** 2 mg/mL	2-12 yrs: 0.20 mg/kg IV (over 5 - 15 sec).
Mometasone Furoate	ELOCON	Corticosteroid	**Cream, Oint & Lotion:** 0.1%	Apply a thin film to affected areas once daily.
Montelukast Sodium	SINGULAIR	Antiasthmatic	**Chewable Tab:** 5 mg **Tab:** 10 mg	6-14 yrs: 5 mg daily po, taken in the PM.
Morphine Sulfate (C-II)		Opioid Analgesic	**Inj:** 0.5 to 15 mg/mL	0.1 - 0.2 mg/kg (up to 15 mg) q 2 - 4 h SC, IM or IV.
Mupirocin	BACTROBAN	Antibacterial	**Oint:** 2%	Apply a small amount to affected area tid.

GENERIC NAME	COMMON TRADE NAMES	THERAPEUTIC CATEGORY	PREPARATIONS	COMMON PEDIATRIC DOSAGE
Nafcillin Sodium	UNIPEN	Antibacterial	Cpsl: 250 mg	**Scarlet Fever and Pneumonia:** 25 mg/kg/day po in 4 divided doses. **Staphylococcal Infections:** 50 mg/kg/day po in 4 divided doses. **Streptococcal Pharyngitis:** 250 mg tid po.
Nalidixic Acid	NEG-GRAM	Urinary Anti-Infective	Susp: 250 mg/5 mL Cplt: 250, 500 mg; 1 g	**Over 3 mos:** Initially 25 mg/lb/day (55 mg/kg/day) po in 4 equally divided doses. For prolonged therapy, the total daily dose may be reduced to 15 mg/lb/day (33 mg/kg/day).
Naloxone Hydrochloride	NARCAN	Opioid Antagonist	Inj (per mL): 0.02, 0.4 mg	**Neonates:** **Opioid-Induced Depression:** 0.01 mg/kg IV, IM, or SC at 2 - 3 min. intervals. Doses may be repeated in 1 - 2 hours. **Children:** **Opioid Overdose:** 0.01 mg/kg IV, followed by 0.1 mg/kg IV, if necessary. If an IV route is not available, may use IM or SC in divided doses. **Postoperative Opioid Respiratory Depression:** 0.005 - 0.01 mg IV at 2 - 3 min. intervals. Doses may be repeated in 1 - 2 hours.
Naproxen	NAPROSYN	Nonsteroidal Anti-Inflammatory Drug	Susp: 125 mg/5 mL Tab: 250, 375, 500 mg	**Juvenile Arthritis (Over 2 yrs):** 5 mg/kg bid po with the total daily dose not to exceed 15 mg/kg/day.
Nedocromil Sodium	TILADE	Antiasthmatic	Aerosol: 1.75 mg/spray	**6-12 yrs:** 2 inhalations qid at regular intervals.

80

| Nelfinavir Mesylate | VIRACEPT | Antiviral | **Powd:** 50 mg/g **Tab:** 250 mg | **2-13 yrs:** 20 - 30 mg/kg/dose, tid po with a meal or a light snack. By body weight, see the Table below: |

Pediatric Dose to be Administered tid po.

Body Weight		Number of Level 1 g Scoops *	Number of Level Teaspoonfuls *	Number of Tablets
kg	lbs			
7.5 to < 8.5	15.5 to < 18.5	4	1	-
8.5 to < 10.5	18.5 to < 23	5	1.25	-
10.5 to < 12	23 to < 26.5	6	1.5	-
12 to < 14	26.5 to < 31	7	1.75	-
14 to < 16	31 to < 35	8	2	-
16 to < 18	35 to < 39.5	9	2.25	-
18 to < 23	39.5 to < 50.5	10	2.5	2
≥ 23	≥ 50.5	15	3.75	3

The oral powder may be mixed with a small amount of water, milk, formula, soy formula, soy milk, or dietary supplements; once mixed, the entire contents must be consumed in order to obtain the full dose. The recommended use period for storage of the product in these media is 6 h.

| Netilmicin Sulfate | NETROMYCIN | Antibacterial | **Inj:** 100 mg/mL | **Neonates (Under 6 weeks):** 4.0 - 6.5 mg/kg/day IV, given as 2.0 - 3.25 mg/kg q 12 h IV.
Infants and Children (6 weeks to 12 yrs): 5.5 - 8.0 mg/kg/day IV, given either as 1.8 to 2.7 mg/kg q 8 h IV or as 2.7 - 4.0 mg/kg q 12 h IV. |

| Nitrofurantoin | FURADANTIN | Urinary Anti-infective, Antibacterial | **Susp:** 25 mg/5 mL | **Over 1 mo:** 5 - 7 mg/kg/24 h po given in 4 divided doses with food. For long-term suppressive therapy, doses as low as 1 mg/kg/24 h po given in single or divided doses may be adequate. |

| Nitrofurantoin Macrocrystals | MACRODANTIN | Urinary Anti-infective, Antibacterial | **Cpsl:** 25, 50, 100 mg | **Over 1 mo:** 5 - 7 mg/kg/day in 4 divided doses po with food. |

81

GENERIC NAME	COMMON TRADE NAMES	THERAPEUTIC CATEGORY	PREPARATIONS	COMMON PEDIATRIC DOSAGE
Norfloxacin	CHIBROXIN	Antibacterial	Ophth Solution: 0.3%	Over 1 yr: 1 - 2 drops into the eye(s) qid for up to 7 days.
Nystatin	MYCOSTATIN	Antifungal	Pastilles: 200,000 Units	200,000 - 400,000 Units 4 or 5 times daily po. Allow to dissolve slowly in the mouth. Continued dosage regimen for at least 48 h after oral symptoms disappear; treatment may continue for as long as 14 days.
			Susp: 100,000 Units/mL	Infants: 200,000 Units (2 mL) qid po (1 mL in in each side of the mouth). Children: 400,000 - 600,000 Units (4 - 6 mL) qid po (1/2 of dose in each side of the mouth).
			Tab: 500,000 Units	Children: 500,000 Units qid po.
			Cream: 100,000 Units/g	Apply liberally to affected areas bid.
			Powd: 100,000 Units/g	Apply to candidal lesions bid or tid.
Ofloxacin	OCUFLOX	Antibacterial	Ophth Solution: 0.3%	Bacterial Conjunctivitis (Over 1 yr): Days 1 and 2: 1 - 2 drops in affected eye(s) q 2 - 4 h. Days 3 to 7: 1 - 2 drops in affected eyes qid. Bacterial Corneal Ulcer (Over 1 yr): Days 1 and 2: 1 - 2 drops in affected eye(s) q 30 min while awake. Awaken at approx. 4 and 6 h after retiring and instill 1 - 2 drops. Days 3 to 7 or 9: 1 - 2 drops in affected eye(s) hourly while awake.
	FLOXIN OTIC		Otic Solution: 0.3%	1-12 yrs: 5 drops into affected ear(s) bid.
Olopatadine Hydrochloride	PATANOL	Antihistamine	Ophth Solution: 0.1%	Over 3 yrs: 1 - 2 drops in each affected eye bid at an interval of 6 - 8 h.

82

Ondansetron Hydrochloride	ZOFRAN	Antiemetic	**Tab:** 4, 8 mg **Solution:** 4 mg/5 mL	**4-12 yrs:** Administer first dose (4 mg po) 30 minutes before the start of emetogenic chemotherapy, with subsequent doses 4 and 8 hours after the first dose. Then, 4 mg tid po for 1 to 2 days after completion of chemotherapy.
			Inj: 2 mg/mL	**4-18 yrs:** Three 0.15 mg/kg doses IV: the first dose is infused over 15 min. beginning 30 minutes before the start of emetogenic chemotherapy. Subsequent doses are administered 4 and 8 h after the first dose.
Oxacillin Sodium	BACTOCILL	Antibacterial	**Cpsl:** 250, 500 mg	**Mild to Moderate Infections of the Skin, Soft Tissue or Upper Respiratory Tract:** 50 mg/kg/day po in divided doses for a minimum of 5 days. **Serious or Life-Threatening Infections:** After initial parenteral treatment, 100 mg/kg/day po in equally divided doses q 4 - 6 h.
			Powd for Inj: 250, 500 mg; 1, 2, 4 g	**Neonates (Birth - 7 days) and** **Under 2 kg:** 50 mg/kg/day in divided doses q 12 h IV. **Over 2 kg:** 75 mg/kg/day in divided doses q 8 h IV. **Neonates (Over 7 days) and** **Under 2 kg:** 100 mg/kg/day in divided doses q 8 h IV. **Over 2 kg:** 150 mg/kg/day in divided doses q 6 h IV. **Mild to Moderate Upper Respiratory and Local Skin and Soft Tissue Infections:** **Children Under 40 kg:** 50 mg/kg/day in equally divided doses q 6 h IM or IV. **Children Over 40 kg:** 250 - 500 mg q 4 - 6 h IM or IV.

[Continued on the next page]

GENERIC NAME	COMMON TRADE NAMES	THERAPEUTIC CATEGORY	PREPARATIONS	COMMON PEDIATRIC DOSAGE
Oxacillin Sodium [Continued]				**Severe Lower Respiratory or Disseminated Infections:** **Children Under 40 kg:** 100 mg/kg/day in equally divided doses q 6 h IM or IV. **Children Over 40 kg:** 1 g q 4 - 6 h IM or IV.
Oxamniquine	VANSIL	Anthelmintic	Cpsl: 250 mg	10 mg/kg bid po with food and with 2 to 8 hours between doses.
Oxiconazole Nitrate	OXISTAT	Antifungal	Cream & Lotion: 1%	*Tinea pedis, T. corporis,* and *T. cruris:* Apply to affected areas once daily or bid for 2 - 4 weeks.
Oxtriphylline		Bronchodilator	Tab: 100, 200 mg	**1-9 yrs:** 7.8 mg/kg po, followed by 6.2 mg/kg q 6 h po. **9-16 yrs:** 7.8 mg/kg po, followed by 4.7 mg/kg q 6 h po.
	CHOLEDYL SA		Sustained-Action Tab: 400, 600 mg	Therapy should be initiated and daily dosage requirements are established using a nonsustained-action form of oxtriphylline. If the total daily dosage of the nonsustained preparation is 1200 mg, then 600 mg of CHOLEDYL SA may be used bid. Similarly, if the total daily dosage is 800 mg, then 400 mg of CHOLEDYL SA may be used bid.
Oxybutynin Chloride	DITROPAN	Urinary Antispasmodic	Syrup: 5 mg/5 mL Tab: 5 mg	**Over 5 yrs:** 5 mg bid po (Maximum: 5 mg tid po).
Oxymetazoline Hydrochloride	AFRIN 12 HOUR, NTZ	Nasal Decongestant	Nasal Solution: 0.05%	**6-12 yrs:** Apply 2 - 3 drops in each nostril bid, morning and evening.
			Nasal Spray: 0.05%	**6-12 yrs:** Spray 2 - 3 times into each nostril bid, morning and evening.

	CHERACOL NASAL, DRISTAN 12-HOUR, 4-WAY LONG LASTING, NEO-SYNEPHRINE MAXIMUM STRENGTH, NOSTRILLA LONG ACTING, VICKS SINEX 12 HOUR		**Nasal Spray:** 0.05%	**6-12 yrs:** Spray 2 - 3 times into each nostril bid, morning and evening.
Oxytetracycline Hydrochloride	VISINE L.R.	Ocular Decongestant	**Ophth Solution:** 0.025%	**Over 6 yrs:** 1 - 2 drops in the affected eye(s) q 6 h.
	TERRAMYCIN	Antibacterial	**Cpsl:** 250 mg	**Over 8 yrs:** 25 - 50 mg/kg/day po in divided doses q 6 h.
Pancuronium Bromide	PAVULON	Neuromuscular Blocker	**Inj (per mL):** 1, 2 mg	**Birth - 1 mo:** 0.02 mg/kg IV as a test dose. **Over 1 mo:** 0.04 - 0.1 mg/kg IV; later, incremental doses starting at 0.01 mg/kg may be used.
Paromomycin Sulfate	HUMATIN	Amebicide	**Cpsl:** 250 mg (of paromomycin base)	**Intestinal Amebiasis:** 25 - 35 mg/kg/day po in 3 divided doses with meals for 5 - 10 days.
Pemoline (C-IV)	CYLERT	CNS Stimulant	**Chewable Tab:** 37.5 mg **Tab:** 18.75, 37.5, 75 mg	**Attention Deficit Disorder (Over 6 yrs):** Starting dose is 37.5 mg/day po. Gradually increase daily dose by 18.75 mg at 1 week intervals until the desired response is obtained. Maximum: 112.5 mg.
Penicillin G Benzathine	BICILLIN L-A	Antibacterial	**Inj (per mL):** 300,000; 600,000 Units	**Streptococcal Upper Respiratory Infections (e.g., Pharyngitis):** **Infants & Children under 60 lb:** 300,000 to 600,000 Units in one single dose IM. **Older Children:** 900,000 Units in one single dose IM. **Congenital Syphilis:** **Under 2 yrs:** 50,000 Units/kg IM. **2-12 yrs:** Adjust dosage based on adult dose (2,400,000 Units IM).

85

GENERIC NAME	COMMON TRADE NAMES	THERAPEUTIC CATEGORY	PREPARATIONS	COMMON PEDIATRIC DOSAGE
Penicillin V Potassium	PEN-VEE K	Antibacterial	Tab: 250, 500 mg Powd for Solution (per 5 mL): 125, 250 mg	Under 12 yrs: 15 - 56 mg/kg/day in 3 - 6 divided doses po.
Pentamidine Isethionate	PENTAM 300	Antiprotozoal	Powd for Inj: 300 mg	4 mg/kg once daily IM or IV (over 60 minutes) for 14 days.
Pentobarbital Sodium (C-II)	NEMBUTAL SODIUM	Sedative - Hypnotic	Inj: 50 mg/mL	2 - 6 mg/kg IM as a single dose. Maximum: 100 mg.
			Elixir: 20 mg/5 mL (18% alcohol) Cpsl: 50, 100 mg	Preoperative Sedation: 2 - 6 mg/kg daily po. Maximum: 100 mg.
			Suppos: 30, 60, 120, 200 mg	Sedation: dose rectally by age - 2-12 mos (10-20 lbs): one 30 mg suppository. 1-4 yrs (20-40 lbs): one 30 mg or 60 mg suppository. 5-12 yrs (40-80 lbs): one 60 mg suppository. 12-14 yrs (80-110 lbs): one 60 mg or one 120 mg suppository.
Permethrin	ELIMITE	Scabicide	Cream: 5%	Over 2 mos: Throughly massage into skin from the head to the soles of the feet. Wash off (bath or shower) after 8 - 14 h. Infants should be treated on the scalp, temple, and forehead.
	NIX		Liquid: 1%	Over 2 mos: Shampoo hair, rinse with water and towel dry. Saturate the hair and scalp (especially behind the ears and on the nape of the neck); allow solution to remain for no longer than 10 mins before rinsing off with water. If live lice are seen 7 days or more after the first application, a second treatment should be given.

86

Phenindamine Tartrate	NOLAHIST	Antihistamine	Tab: 25 mg	6-12 yrs: 12.5 mg q 4 - 6 h po, not to exceed 3 tablets in 24 h.
Phenobarbital (C-IV)		Pre-Op. Sedative, Anticonvulsant	Elixir: 20 mg/5 mL (alcohol) Tab: 15, 30, 60, 100 mg	Sedation: 1 - 3 mg/kg po. Convulsions: 3 - 6 mg/kg/day in divided doses q 12 h po.
Phenobarbital Sodium (C-IV)		Pre-Op. Sedative, Anticonvulsant	Inj (per mL): 30, 60, 65, 130 mg	Preoperative Sedation: 1 - 3 mg/kg IM or IV. Convulsions: 4 - 6 mg/kg/day for 7 - 10 days to blood levels of 10 - 15 µg/mL or 10 - 15 mg/kg/day IM or IV.
Phenol	CEPASTAT	Local Anesthetic (Oral)	Lozenge (Cherry Flavor): 14.5 mg	6-12 yrs: Dissolve 1 slowly in the mouth. May repeat q 2 h, not to exceed 20 lozenges per day.
			Lozenge (Extra Strength): 29 mg	6-12 yrs: Dissolve 1 slowly in the mouth. May repeat q 2 h, not to exceed 10 lozenges per day.
	VICKS CHILDREN'S CHLORASEPTIC		Spray: 0.5%	Over 2 yrs: Spray 5 times daily directly on throat or affected area and swallow. Repeat q 2 h prn.
	CHLORASEPTIC SORE THROAT SPRAY & GARGLE		Solution (with & without sprayer): 1.4%	2-12 yrs: Spray 3 times directly into throat or affected area and swallow. 6-12 yrs: Gargle or swish around in mouth 10 mL for at least 15 seconds, then spit out. Use every 2 hours.
Phentolamine Mesylate	REGITINE	Antihypertensive	Powd for Inj: 5 mg	Preoperative: 1 mg IM or IV, 1 - 2 h before surgery, and repeated if necessary. During Surgery: 1 mg IV as required.

87

GENERIC NAME	COMMON TRADE NAMES	THERAPEUTIC CATEGORY	PREPARATIONS	COMMON PEDIATRIC DOSAGE
Phenylephrine Hydrochloride	NEO-SYNEPHRINE	Nasal Decongestant	**Nasal Solution:** 0.125, 0.25, 0.5%	**Infants:** 1 drop in each nostril q 2 - 4 h (of the 0.125% solution). **2-6 yrs:** 1 - 2 drops in each nostril q 4 h (of the 0.25% solution). **6-12 yrs:** 2 - 3 drops in each nostril q 4 h (of the 0.25% solution).
	NEO-SYNEPHRINE, NOSTRIL		**Nasal Spray:** 0.25, 0.5%	**2-6 yrs:** 1 - 2 sprays in each nostril q 4 h (of the 0.25% solution). **6-12 yrs:** 2 - 3 sprays in each nostril q 4 h (of the 0.25% solution).
	NEO-SYNEPHRINE	Sympathomimetic	**Inj:** 10 mg/mL (1%)	**Hypotension During Spinal Anesthesia:** 0.5 - 1 mg per 25 lbs SC or IM.
Phenylpropanolamine Hydrochloride	PROPAGEST	Decongestant	**Tab:** 25 mg	**6-12 yrs:** 12.5 mg q 4 h po.
Phenytoin	DILANTIN-125 DILANTIN INFATAB	Antiepileptic	**Susp (per 5 mL):** 125 mg **Chewable Tab:** 50 mg	**Initial:** 5 mg/kg/day in 2 or 3 equally divided doses po. Maximum: 300 mg daily. **Maintenance:** 4 - 8 mg/kg po. Children over 6 years old may require the minimum adult dose of 300 mg/day.
Phenytoin Sodium	DILANTIN	Antiepileptic	**Cpsl:** 30, 100 mg	**Initial:** 5 mg/kg/day in 2 or 3 equally divided doses po. Maximum: 300 mg daily. **Maintenance:** 4 - 8 mg/kg po. Children over 6 yrs old may require the minimum adult dose of 300 mg/day.
	DILANTIN		**Inj:** 50 mg/mL	**Status Epilepticus:** A loading dose of 15 - 20 mg/kg slow IV (at a rate not exceeding 1 - 3 mg/kg/min).
Phytonadione	AQUA-MEPHYTON	Vitamin K$_1$	**Inj (per mL):** 2, 10 mg	**Hemorrhagic Disease in Newborns:** **Prophylaxis:** 0.5 - 1 mg IM within 1 hour after birth. **Treatment:** 1 mg SC or IM.

Pipecuronium Bromide	ARDUAN	Neuromuscular Blocker	Powd for Inj: 10 mg	**Endotracheal Intubation:** 3-12 mos: 70 - 85 μg/kg IV (same as the adult dosage). 1-14 yrs: (children may be less sensitive than adults). **Maintenance:** 3-12 mos: 10 - 15 μg/kg IV (same as the adult dosage). 1-14 yrs: (children may be less sensitive than adults).
Povidone-Iodine	BETADINE FIRST AID CREAM	Antiseptic	Cream: 5%	Apply directly to the affected area prn.
	BETADINE		Oint: 10%	Apply directly to affected area prn.
			Solution: 10%	Apply directly to affected area prn.
	BETADINE SKIN CLEANSER		Liquid: 7.5%	Wet the skin and apply a sufficient amount to work up a rich golden lather. Allow lather to remain for about 3 min; rinse thoroughly with water. Repeat bid - tid prn.
Praziquantel	BILTRICIDE	Anthelmintic	Tab: 600 mg	**Schistosomiasis (Over 4 yrs):** 20 mg/kg po tid for 1 day. **Clonorchiasis and Opisthorchiasis (Over 4 yrs):** 25 mg/kg po tid for 1 day.
Prednicarbate	DERMATOP	Corticosteroid	Cream: 0.1%	**Over 1 yr:** Apply a thin film to skin bid. Rub in gently. Do not use for more than 3 weeks.
Prednisolone Sodium Phosphate	PEDIAPRED	Corticosteroid	Liquid: 6.7 mg/5 mL (equivalent to 5 mg of prednisolone base/5 mL)	Initial dose may vary from 5 to 60 mg po per day. Dose requirements are variable and must be individualized based on the disease and the patient's response.
Prednisone	DELTASONE LIQUID PRED	Corticosteroid	Tab: 2.5, 5, 10, 20, 50 mg Syrup: 5 mg/5 mL (5% alcohol)	Initial dose may vary from 5 to 60 mg po per day. Dose requirements are variable and must be individualized based on the disease and the patient's response.

GENERIC NAME	COMMON TRADE NAMES	THERAPEUTIC CATEGORY	PREPARATIONS	COMMON PEDIATRIC DOSAGE
Primaquine Phosphate	PRIMAQUINE PHOSPHATE	Antimalarial	Tab: 26.3 mg (equal to 15 mg of primaquine base)	0.3 mg/kg/day po for 14 days.
Primidone	MYSOLINE	Antiepileptic	Susp: 250 mg/5 mL Tab: 50, 250 mg	**Under 8 yrs:** 50 mg hs po (for 3 days); 50 mg bid po (for 3 days); 100 mg bid po (for 3 days); then 125 - 250 mg tid po. **Over 8 yrs:** 100 - 125 mg hs po (for 3 days); 100 - 125 mg bid po (for 3 days); 100 - 125 mg tid po (for 3 days); then 250 mg tid po.
Probenecid		Penicillin / Cephalosporin Adjunct	Tab: 500 mg	**2-14 yrs:** 25 mg/kg po, followed by 10 mg/kg qid po (Maximum: the adult dose of 500 mg qid po).
Procarbazine Hydrochloride	MATULANE	Antineoplastic	Cpsl: 50 mg	50 mg/m^2/day po for 1 week; then maintain the dosage at 100 mg/m^2/day until maximum response occurs or until leukopenia or thrombocytopenia occurs. Then maintain dose at 50 mg/m^2/day.
Prochlorperazine	COMPAZINE	Antiemetic, Antipsychotic	Suppos: 2.5, 5 mg	**Severe Nausea and Vomiting (Over 2 yrs and by weight):** **20-29 lbs:** 2.5 mg rectally 1 or 2 times daily. **30-39 lbs:** 2.5 mg rectally bid or tid. **40-85 lbs:** 2.5 mg rectally tid or 5 mg rectally bid. **Psychosis:** **2-5 yrs:** Initially 2.5 mg rectally bid or tid (maximum: 10 mg on the first day). Then increase dosage according to patient's response. Maximum: 20 mg/day. **6-12 yrs:** Initially 2.5 mg rectally bid or tid (maximum: 10 mg on the first day). Then increase dosage according to patient's response. Maximum: 25 mg/day.

Prochlorperazine Edisylate	COMPAZINE	Antiemetic, Antipsychotic	Syrup: 5 mg/5 mL	**Severe Nausea and Vomiting (Over 2 yrs):** and by weight - **20-29 lbs:** 2.5 mg po 1 or 2 times daily. **30-39 lbs:** 2.5 mg po bid or tid. **40-85 lbs:** 2.5 mg po tid or 5 mg po bid. **Psychosis:** **2-5 yrs:** Initially 2.5 mg po bid or tid (maximum: 10 mg on the first day). Then increase dosage according to patient's response. Maximum: 20 mg/day. **6-12 yrs:** Initially 2.5 mg po bid or tid (maximum: 10 mg on the first day). Then increase dosage according to patient's response. Maximum: 25 mg/day.
			Inj: 5 mg/mL	**Severe Nausea and Vomiting (Over 2 yrs):** 0.06 mg/lb by deep IM (single dose). **Psychosis (2-12 yrs):** 0.06 mg/lb by deep IM. Control is usually obtained with one dose.
Prochlorperazine Maleate	COMPAZINE	Antiemetic, Antipsychotic	Tab: 5, 10 mg	Same dosages as for COMPAZINE Syrup above.
Promethazine Hydrochloride	PHENERGAN	Sedative, Antiemetic, Antihistamine	Syrup (PLAIN): 6.25 mg/5 mL (7% alcohol) Syrup (FORTIS): 25 mg/5 mL (1.5% alcohol) Tab: 12.5, 25, 50 mg Suppos: 12.5, 25, 50 mg	**Over 2 yrs:** **Sedation:** 12.5 - 25 mg hs po or rectally. **Allergy:** 6.25 - 12.5 mg tid po or 25 mg hs po. **Motion Sickness:** 12.5 - 25 mg po or rectally. **Nausea & Vomiting:** 0.5 mg/lb po or rectally (average dose is 25 mg) q 4 - 6 h prn.
			Inj (per mL): 25, 50 mg	**Nausea & Vomiting (Over 2 yrs):** When oral medication cannot be tolerated. 0.5 mg/lb q 4 - 6 h IM (e.g., 12.5 - 25 mg) can be used.
Propranolol Hydrochloride	INDERAL	Antihypertensive	Tab: 10, 20, 40, 60, 80 mg	Initially, 1.0 mg/kg/day in 2 equally divided doses po. The usual dosage range is 2 - 4 mg/kg/day in 2 equally divided doses po.

GENERIC NAME	COMMON TRADE NAMES	THERAPEUTIC CATEGORY	PREPARATIONS	COMMON PEDIATRIC DOSAGE
Propylhexedrine	BENZEDREX INHALER	Nasal Decongestant	**Inhalant Tube:** delivers 0.4 to 0.5 mg/800 mL of air	**6-12 yrs:** 2 inhalations in each nostril not more often than q 2 h.
Propylthiouracil		Antithyroid Agent	**Tab:** 50 mg	**6-10 yrs:** Initially, 50 - 150 mg daily po in divided doses q 8 h; the maintenance dose is usually 1/3 to 2/3 of initial daily dose, but should be determined by the patient's response. **Over 10 yrs:** Initially, 150 - 300 mg daily po in divided doses q 8 h; the maintenance dose is usually 1/3 to 2/3 of initial daily dose, but should be determined by the patient's response.
Pseudoephedrine Hydrochloride	PEDIACARE INFANT'S ORAL DECONGESTANT	Nasal Decongestant	**Solution (Drops):** 7.5 mg/0.8 mL	**Birth - 3 mos (6-11 lbs):** 0.4 mL q 4 - 6 h po. **4-11 mos (12-17 lbs):** 0.8 mL q 4 - 6 h po. **12-23 mos (18-23 lbs):** 1.2 mL q 4 - 6 h po. **2-3 yrs (24-35 lbs):** 1.6 mL q 4 - 6 h po.
	SUDAFED CHILDREN'S NASAL DECONGESTANT		**Liquid:** 15 mg/5 mL	**2-5 yrs:** 5 mL q 4 - 6 h po. **6-12 yrs:** 10 mL q 4 - 6 h po.
			Chewable Tab: 15 mg	**2-6 yrs:** Chew 1 tab q 4 - 6 h po. **6-12 yrs:** Chew 2 tabs q 4 - 6 h po.
	DORCOL CHILDREN'S DECONGESTANT		**Liquid:** 15 mg/5 mL	**3-12 mos:** 3 drops/kg q 4 - 6 h po. **12-24 mos:** 7 drops (0.2 mL)/kg q 4 - 6 h po. **2-5 yrs (or 25-45 lbs):** 5 mL q 4 - 6 h po. **6-12 yrs (or 46-85 lbs):** 10 mL q 4 - 6 h po.
	TRIAMINIC AM DECONGESTANT FORMULA		**Liquid:** 15 mg/5 mL	**3-12 mos (12-17 lbs):** 1.25 mL q 6 h po. **12-24 mos (18-23 lbs):** 2.5 mL q 6 h po. **2-5 yrs (24-47 lbs):** 5 mL q 4 - 6 h po. **6-12 yrs (48-95 lbs):** 10 mL q 4 - 6 h po.
	SUDAFED		**Tab:** 30 mg	**6-12 yrs:** 30 mg q 4 - 6 h po.

Psyllium	METAMUCIL	Bulk Laxative	Powder (Regular): 3.4 g per rounded teaspoonful Powder (Flavored): 3.4 g per tablespoonful	6-12 yrs: 1/2 rounded teaspoonful (Regular) or tablespoonful (Flavored) in 8 oz. of liquid 1 to 3 times daily po.
			Wafer: 3.4 g	6-12 yrs: 1 wafer with 8 oz. of liquid 1 - 3 times daily po.
	PERDIEM FIBER THERAPY		Granules: 4.03 g/rounded teaspoonful (6.0 g)	7-11 yrs: 1 rounded teaspoonful 1 - 2 times daily po with 8 oz. of a cool beverage.
Psyllium Hydrophilic Mucilloid	FIBERALL	Bulk Laxative	Powder: 3.4 g/rounded teaspoonful (5.0 - 5.9 g)	6-11 yrs: 1/2 rounded teaspoonful in 8 oz. of liquid 1 - 3 times daily po.
			Wafer: 3.4 g	6-11 yrs: 1/2 - 1 wafer with 8 oz. of liquid 1 to 3 times daily po.
	EFFER-SYLLIUM		Powder: 3 g/rounded teaspoonful Packet: 3 g	Over 6 yrs: 1 level teaspoonful, or 1/2 packet, in 1/2 glass of water hs po.
	KONSYL FOR KIDS		Powder: 2 g/rounded teaspoonful (7.0 g)	6-12 yrs: 1 rounded teaspoonful in 8 oz. of cool liquid 1 - 3 times daily po.
	KONSYL		Powder: 6 g/rounded teaspoonful (6.0 g)	6-12 yrs: 1/2 rounded teaspoonful in 8 oz. of liquid 1 - 3 times daily po.
	KONSYL-D		Powder: 3.4 g/rounded teaspoonful (6.5 g) [contains added dextrose]	6-12 yrs: 1/2 rounded teaspoonful in 8 oz. of liquid 1 - 3 times daily po.
	KONSYL-ORANGE		Powder: 3.4 g/rounded teaspoonful (12.0 g)	6-12 yrs: 1/2 rounded teaspoonful in 8 oz. of liquid 1 - 3 times daily po.

93

GENERIC NAME	COMMON TRADE NAMES	THERAPEUTIC CATEGORY	PREPARATIONS	COMMON PEDIATRIC DOSAGE
	SERUTAN		Granules: 2.5 g/heaping teaspoonful	**6-12 yrs:** 1/2 - 1-1/2 heaping teaspoonfuls on cereal or other food 1 - 3 times daily po. Drink at least 8 oz. of liquid with the food.
			Powder: 3.4 g/heaping teaspoonful	**6-12 yrs:** 1/2 heaping teaspoonful in 8 oz. of water 1 - 3 times daily po, preferably with meals.
	SYLLACT		Powder: 3.3 g/rounded teaspoonful	**6-12 yrs:** 1/2 - 1 rounded teaspoonful in 8 oz. of liquid 1 - 3 times daily po.
Pyrantel Pamoate	PIN-X, ANTIMINTH	Anthelmintic	Liquid: 144 mg/mL (equivalent to 50 mg/mL of pyrantel)	**Over 2 yrs:** 5 mg/lb (to a maximum of 1 g) as a single dose po. Dosage by weight is shown below: **25-37 lbs:** 2.5 mL **38-62 lbs:** 5 mL **63-87 lbs:** 7.5 mL **88-112 lbs:** 10 mL **113-137 lbs:** 12.5 mL **138-162 lbs:** 15 mL
	REESE'S PINWORM MEDICINE		Liquid: 144 mg/mL (equivalent to 50 mg/mL of pyrantel) Cpsl: 180 mg (equivalent to 62.5 mg of pyrantel)	**Over 2 yrs:** 5 mg/lb (to a maximum of 1 g) as a single dose po.
Pyrazinamide		Tuberculostatic	Tab: 500 mg	15 - 30 mg/kg once daily po. Maximum: 2 g/day.
Pyrimethamine	DARAPRIM	Antimalarial	Tab: 25 mg	**Chemoprophylaxis:** **Under 4 yrs:** 6.25 mg once weekly po. **4-10 yrs:** 12.5 mg once weekly po. **Over 10 yrs:** 25 mg once weekly po.
Quinine Sulfate		Antimalarial	Cpsl: 200, 260, 325 mg Tab: 260 mg	10 mg/kg q 8 h po for 5 - 7 days.

94

Ribavirin	VIRAZOLE	Antiviral	**Powder for Aerosol:** 6 g (20 mg/mL after reconstitution)	Reconstitute with 300 mL water. Treatment with the Viratek Small Particle Aerosol Generator (SPAG) for 12 - 18 h/day for 3 - 7 days using an infant oxygen hood.
Rifampin	RIFADIN RIFADIN I.V.	Tuberculostatic	**Cpsl:** 150, 300 mg **Powd for Inj:** 600 mg	10 - 20 mg/kg once daily po (1 hour before or 2 hours after a meal) or IV, not to exceed 600 mg/day.
Rimantadine Hydrochloride	FLUMADINE	Antiviral	**Syrup:** 50 mg/5 mL **Tab:** 100 mg	**Prophylaxis:** **Under 10 yrs:** 5 mg/kg once daily po, not to exceed 150 mg. **Over 10 yrs:** Use the adult dose of 100 mg bid po.
Ritonavir	NORVIR	Antiviral	**Solution:** 80 mg/mL **Cpsl:** 100 mg	**Over 2 yrs:** Use in combination with nucleoside analogues. Initially 250 mg/m² bid po with food. Increase at 2 - 3 day intervals by increments of 50 mg/m² bid po as tolerated to a target dose of 400 mg/m² bid with food. Maximum: 600 mg bid with food.
Rocuronium Bromide	ZEMURON	Neuromuscular Blocker	**Inj:** 10 mg/mL	**3 mos - 12 yrs:** Initially, 0.6 mg/kg IV with halothane anesthesia have been used for intubation; maintenance doses of 0.075 to 0.125 mg/kg IV have provided good muscle relaxation.
Salicylic Acid	DUOFILM PATCH FOR KIDS	Keratolytic	**Patch:** 40%	**Over 2 yrs:** Wash affected area. May soak wart in warm water for 5 min; dry area thoroughly. Apply patch. Repeat procedure q 48 h prn (until wart is removed) for up to 12 weeks.
Scopolamine Hydrobromide	ISOPTO HYOSCINE	Mydriatic - Cycloplegic	**Ophth Solution:** 0.25%	**Refraction:** Instill 1 - 2 drops in the eye(s) 1 hour before refracting. **Uveitis:** Instill 1 - 2 drops in the eye(s) up to

GENERIC NAME	COMMON TRADE NAMES	THERAPEUTIC CATEGORY	PREPARATIONS	COMMON PEDIATRIC DOSAGE
Secobarbital Sodium (C-II)		Sedative - Hypnotic	Inj: 50 mg/mL	**Preoperative Sedation:** 4 - 5 mg/kg IM.
Senna Concentrate	FLETCHER'S CASTORIA FOR CHILDREN	Stimulant Laxative	Liquid: 33.3 mg/mL (3.5% alcohol)	**1-6 mos:** 1.25 - 2.5 mL hs po. **7-12 mos:** 2.5 - 5 mL hs po. **1-5 yrs:** 5 - 10 mL hs po. **6-12 yrs:** 10 - 15 mL hs po.
	SENOKOT		Syrup: 218 mg/5 mL (7% alcohol) [8.8 mg of sennosides/5 mL]	**2-6 yrs:** 2.5 - 3.75 mL po. Maximum: 3.75 mL bid po. **6-12 yrs:** 5 - 7.5 mL hs po. Maximum: 7.5 mL bid po.
			Tab: 187 mg [8.6 mg of sennosides]	**2-6 yrs:** 1/2 tab once daily po. Maximum: 1 tab bid po. **6-12 yrs:** 1 tab once daily po. Maximum: 2 tabs bid po.
			Granules: 326 mg/tsp. [15 mg of sennosides per tsp.]	**2-6 yrs:** 1/4 teaspoonful once daily po. Maximum: 1/2 teaspoonful bid po. **6-12 yrs:** 1/2 teaspoonful once daily po. Maximum: 1 teaspoonful bid po.
	SENOKOTXTRA		Tab: 374 mg [17 mg of sennosides]	**6-12 yrs:** 1/2 tab once daily po. Maximum: 1 tablet bid po.
Sennosides	EX-LAX	Stimulant Laxative	Chewable Tab: 15 mg	**6-12 yrs:** Chew 1 tab once daily or bid.
	EX-LAX, REGULAR STRENGTH		Pill: 15 mg	**6-12 yrs:** 1 pill once daily or bid with a glass of water.
	EX-LAX, MAXIMUM STRENGTH		Pill: 25 mg	**6-12 yrs:** 1 pill once daily or bid with a glass of water.

Sertraline Hydrochloride	ZOLOFT	Drug for Obsessive-Compulsive Disorder	Tab: 25, 50, 100 mg	**6-12 yrs:** Initially 25 mg once daily po. May increase at 1 week intervals. Maximum: 100 mg daily.
Simethicone	INFANTS' MYLICON, PHAZYME	Antiflatulent	**Solution (Drops):** 40 mg/0.6 mL	**Under 2 yrs:** 0.3 mL (20 mg) qid pc and hs po. **2-12 yrs:** 0.6 mL (40 mg) qid pc and hs po.
	GAS-X		**Liquid:** 50 mg/5 mL	**2-12 yrs:** 5 mL po pc & hs.
Sodium Fluoride	LURIDE, PEDIAFLOR	Fluoride Supplement	**Solution (Drops):** 1.1 mg/mL (equivalent to 0.5 mg/mL of fluoride)	**Less Than 0.3 ppm Fluoride in Drinking Water:** **6 mos - 3 yrs:** 1/2 dropperful (0.25 mg) daily po. **3-6 yrs:** 1 dropperful (0.5 mg) daily po. **6-16 yrs:** 2 dropperfuls (1.0 mg) daily po. **0.3 to 0.6 ppm Fluoride in Drinking Water:** **3-6 yrs:** 1/2 dropperful (0.25 mg) daily po. **6-16 yrs:** 1 dropperful (0.5 mg) daily po.
	LURIDE LOZI-TABS LURIDE SF	Fluoride Supplement	**Chewable Tab:** 0.25, 0.5, 1 mg **Chewable Tab:** 0.25 mg	**Less Than 0.3 ppm Fluoride in Drinking Water:** **6 mos - 3 yrs:** 0.25 mg daily po. **3-6 yrs:** 0.5 mg daily po. **6-16 yrs:** 1.0 mg daily po. **0.3 to 0.6 ppm Fluoride in Drinking Water:** **3-6 yrs:** 0.25 mg daily po. **6-16 yrs:** 0.5 mg daily po.
Sodium Nitroprusside		Antihypertensive	**Inj:** 50 mg (in 1 L D_5W)	The average effective IV infusion rate is about 3 μg/kg/min. At this rate, some patients will become dangerously hypotensive. Begin IV infusion at a very low rate (0.3 μg/kg/min), with gradual upward titration every few minutes until the desired effect is achieved or the maximum rate (10 μg/kg/min) has been reached.

GENERIC NAME	COMMON TRADE NAMES	THERAPEUTIC CATEGORY	PREPARATIONS	COMMON PEDIATRIC DOSAGE
Sodium Polystyrene Sulfonate	KAYEXALATE	Potassium-Removing Resin	**Powder:** 10 - 12 g/heaping teaspoonful.	Use as a guide that each g of resin exchanges approximately 1 mEq of potassium (in vivo). Give each dose as a suspension in a liquid.
	SODIUM POLYSTYRENE SULFONATE SUSP.		**Susp:** 15 g/60 mL (0.1% alcohol)	Use as a guide that each g of resin exchanges approximately 1 mEq of potassium (in vivo).
Spironolactone	ALDACTONE	Diuretic	**Tab:** 25, 50, 100 mg	1.5 mg/lb/day po in a single or divided doses.
Stavudine	ZERIT	Antiviral	**Powd for Soln:** 1 mg/mL **Cpsl:** 15, 20, 30, 40 mg	**Initial Dosage:** **Under 30 kg:** 2 mg/kg/day (given q 12 h) po. **Equal to or Over 30 kg:** 30 mg twice daily (q 12 h) po. **Dosage Adjustment:** Monitor patients for the development of peripheral neuropathy. If symptoms develop, stop the drug. If the symptoms resolve completely, consider resumption of therapy with half of the above mg dosages.
Streptomycin Sulfate		Tuberculostatic	**Inj:** 1 g/2.5 mL	**Tuberculosis:** either of the following regimens are used. Generally no more than 120 g is given over the course of therapy. 20 - 40 mg/kg daily IM. Maximum: 1 g. 25 - 30 mg/kg two or three times weekly IM. Maximum: 1.5 g.
Succinylcholine Chloride	ANECTINE	Neuromuscular Blocker	**Inj:** 20 mg/mL **Powd for IV Infusion:** 500, 1000 mg	**Endotrachial Intubation:** **Infants and Small Children:** 2 mg/kg IV. **Older Children and Adolescents:** 1 mg/kg IV.

Sulfacetamide Sodium	BLEPH-10 ISOPTO CETAMIDE	Antibacterial	Ophth Solution: 10% Ophth Solution: 15%	**Conjunctivitis or Corneal Ulcer (Over 2 mos):** Initially, 1 - 2 drops into eye(s) q 2 - 3 h. Dosages may be tapered by increasing the time interval between doses as the condition responds. The usual duration of treatment is 7 - 10 days. **Trachoma (Over 2 mos):** 2 drops into eye(s) q 2 h.
	BLEPH-10, CETAMIDE		Ophth Oint: 10%	**Conjunctivitis or Corneal Ulcer (Over 2 mos):** Apply a small amount (about 1/2 in.) into eye(s) q 3 - 4 h & hs. Dosages may be tapered by increasing the time interval between doses as the condition responds. The usual duration of treatment is 7 - 10 days.
	SODIUM SULAMYD		Ophth Solution: 10%	**Conjunctivitis or Corneal Ulcer (Over 2 mos):** 1 - 2 drops into eye(s) q 2 - 3 h during the day, less often at night.
			Ophth Solution: 30%	**Conjunctivitis or Corneal Ulcer (Over 2 mos):** 1 drop into the affected eye(s) q 2 h or less frequently according to the severity of the infection. **Trachoma (Over 2 mos):** 2 drops into eye(s) q 2 h.
			Ophth Oint: 10%	**Conjunctivitis or Corneal Ulcer (Over 2 mos):** Apply a small amount into eye(s) qid & hs.
Sulfadiazine		Antibacterial	Tab: 500 mg	**Usual Infections (Over 2 mos):** 75 mg/kg (or 2 g/m²) po as a loading dose, followed by 150 mg/kg/day (4 g/m²/day) in 4 - 6 divided doses po. Maximum: 6 g/day. **Toxoplasmosis:** **Under 2 mos:** 25 mg/kg/dose qid po. **Over 2 mos:** 25 - 50 mg/kg/dose qid po.

GENERIC NAME	COMMON TRADE NAMES	THERAPEUTIC CATEGORY	PREPARATIONS	COMMON PEDIATRIC DOSAGE
Sulfamethizole	THIOSULFIL FORTE	Antibacterial	**Tab:** 500 mg	**Over 2 mos:** 30 - 45 mg/kg/day po in 4 divided doses.
Sulfamethoxazole	GANTANOL	Antibacterial	**Tab:** 500 mg	**Over 2 mos (Initial):** 50 - 60 mg/kg po. **Over 2 mos (Maintenance):** 25 - 30 mg/kg q 12 h po. Maximum: 75 mg/kg/day.
Sulfasalazine	AZULFIDINE AZULFIDINE-EN	Bowel Anti-Inflammatory Agent	**Tab:** 500 mg **Enteric-Coated Tab:** 500 mg	**Over 2 yrs (Initial):** 40 - 60 mg/kg each day po divided into 3 - 6 doses. **Over 2 yrs (Maintenance):** 30 mg/kg/day po divided into 4 doses.
Sulfisoxazole		Antibacterial	**Tab:** 500 mg	**Over 2 mos (Initial):** 75 mg/kg po. **Over 2 mos (Maintenance):** 150 mg/kg/day (4 g/m²/day) po in 4 - 6 divided doses. Maximum: 6 g/day.
Sulfisoxazole Acetyl		Antibacterial	**Pediatric Susp:** 500 mg/5 mL (0.3% alcohol) **Syrup:** 500 mg/5 mL (0.9% alcohol)	**Over 2 mos:** Initially, 75 mg/kg po; then, 150 mg/kg/day po in 4 - 6 divided doses. Maximum: 6 g per 24 hours.
Tacrolimus	PROGRAF	Immunosuppressant	**Cpsl:** 1, 5 mg **Inj:** 5 mg/mL	0.15 - 0.3 mg/kg/day po in 2 divided doses (q 12 h). Administer initial dose no sooner than 6 h after transplantation. If IV therapy was initiated, begin 8 - 12 h after discontinuing IV therapy. 0.05 - 0.1 mg/kg/day as a continuous IV infusion. Administer initial dose no sooner than 6 h after transplantation. Convert to oral therapy as soon as the patient can tolerate oral dosing.

Tetracaine Hydrochloride	CEPACOL VIRACTIN	Local Anesthetic (Oral)	**Cream & Gel:** 2%	**Over 2 yrs:** Apply to the affected area around lips and mouth up to qid.
	PONTOCAINE	Local Anesthetic (Topical)	**Cream:** 1%	Apply to the affected area prn.
Tetracycline Hydrochloride	SUMYCIN	Antibacterial	**Susp:** 125 mg/5 mL **Cpsl & Tab:** 250, 500 mg	**Over 8 yrs:** 10 - 20 mg/lb/day po divided into 2 or 4 equal doses.
Tetrahydrozoline Hydrochloride	VISINE ORIGINAL	Ocular Decongestant	**Ophth Solution:** 0.05%	**Over 6 yrs:** 1 - 2 drops in affected eye(s) up to qid.
	TYZINE	Nasal Decongestant	**Nasal Solution:** 0.05, 0.1%	**2-6 yrs:** 2 - 3 drops (of the 0.05% solution) in each nostril q 4 - 6 h. **Over 6 yrs:** 2 - 4 drops (of the 0.1% solution) in each nostril q 4 - 6 h.
Theophylline, Anhydrous	AEROLATE	Bronchodilator	**Cpsl:** 65, 130, 260 mg	65 or 130 mg q 12 h po; in severe attacks, 65 or 130 mg q 8 h po.
	ELIXOPHYLLIN		**Elixir:** 80 mg/15 mL (20% alcohol) **Cpsl:** 100, 200 mg	See the Theophylline Table, Section I, p. 158.
	RESPBID		**Sustained-Rel. Tab:** 250, 500 mg	See the Theophylline Table, Section IIA, p. 159.
	SLO-BID		**Extended-Rel. Cpsl:** 50, 75, 100, 125, 200, 300 mg	See the Theophylline Table, Section IIA, p. 159.
	SLO-PHYLLIN		**Syrup:** 80 mg/15 mL **Tab:** 100, 200 mg **Extended-Rel. Cpsl:** 60, 125, 250 mg	See the Theophylline Table, Section I, p. 158. See the Theophylline Table, Section IIA, p. 159.
	THEO-DUR		**Extended-Rel. Tab:** 100, 200, 300, 450 mg	See the Theophylline Table, Section IIB, p. 159.

[Continued on the next page]

101

GENERIC NAME	COMMON TRADE NAMES	THERAPEUTIC CATEGORY	PREPARATIONS	COMMON PEDIATRIC DOSAGE
Theophylline, Anhydrous [Continued]	THEOLAIR		Liquid: 80 mg/15 mL Tab: 125, 250 mg	See the Theophylline Table, Section I, p. 158.
	THEOLAIR-SR		Sustained-Rel. Tab: 200, 250, 300, 500 mg	See the Theophylline Table, Section IIA, p. 159.
Thiabendazole	MINTEZOL	Anthelmintic	Susp: 500 mg/5 mL Chewable Tab: 500 mg	**Strongyloidiasis, Intestinal Roundworms, and Cutaneous Larva Migrans:** 2 doses/day (as below) for 2 successive days po. **Trichinosis:** 2 doses/day (as below) for 2 - 4 successive days po. **Visceral Larva Migrans:** 2 doses/day (as below) for 7 successive days. Dose: 10 mg/lb (over 30 lb).
Thioguanine		Antineoplastic	Tab: 40 mg	Initially, 2 mg/kg daily po. If no improvement occurs after 4 weeks, the dosage may be cautiously increased to 3 mg/kg/day.
Thioridazine	MELLARIL-S	Antipsychotic	Susp (per 5 mL): 25, 100 mg	**2-12 yrs:** 0.5 - 1 mg/kg/day po (maximum: 3 mg/kg/day). For children with moderate disorders, 10 mg bid to tid is the usual starting dose. For hospitalized, severely disturbed, or psychotic children, 25 mg bid to tid is the usual starting dose. Dosage may be increased gradually until optimum therapeutic effect is obtained or the maximum has been reached.
Thioridazine Hydrochloride	MELLARIL	Antipsychotic	Liquid Conc (per mL): 30, (3% alcohol), 100 mg (4.2% (alcohol) Tab: 10, 15, 25, 50, 100, 150, 200 mg	**2-12 yrs:** Same dosage as for MELLARIL-S above.

Thyroid Desiccated	ARMOUR THYROID	Thyroid Hormone	Tab: 15, 30, 60, 90, 120, 180, 240, 300 mg	**Congenital Hypothyroidism:** **Birth - 6 mos:** 4.8 - 6 mg/kg/day po. **6-12 mos:** 3.6 - 4.8 mg/kg/day po. **1-5 yrs:** 3 - 3.6 mg/kg/day po. **6-12 yrs:** 2.4 - 3 mg/kg/day po.
Ticarcillin Disodium	TICAR	Antibacterial	Powd for Inj: 1, 3, 6 g	**Neonates (Birth - 7 days) and** **Under 2 kg:** 75 mg/kg q 12 h IM or by IV infusion. **Over 2 kg:** 75 mg/kg q 8 h IM or by IV infusion. **Neonates (Over 7 days) and** **Under 2 kg:** 75 mg/kg q 8 h IM or by IV infusion. **Over 2 kg:** 100 mg/kg q 8 h IM or by IV infusion. **Older Neonates and Children (Under 40 kg):** **Uncomplicated UTI:** 50 - 100 mg/kg/day in divided doses q 6 - 8 h IM or direct IV. **Complicated UTI:** 150 - 200 mg/kg/day in divided doses q 4 - 6 h by IV infusion. **Septicemia, Respiratory, Intra-Abdominal, Skin and Soft Tissue Infections:** 200 - 300 mg/kg/day in divided doses q 4 - 6 h by IV infusion. **Children (Over 40 kg):** Should receive adult dosages.
Tobramycin	TOBREX	Antibacterial	Ophth Oint: 3 mg/g (0.3%)	**Mild to Moderate Infections:** Apply 1/2 inch ribbon into the affected eye(s) bid - tid. **Severe Infections:** Apply 1/2 inch ribbon into the affected eye(s) q 3 - 4 h until improvement occurs; reduce dosage prior to discontinuation.
			Ophth Solution: 3 mg/mL (0.3%)	**Mild to Moderate Infections:** 1 - 2 drops into the affected eye(s) q 4 h. **Severe Infections:** 2 drops into the affected eye(s) hourly until improvement occurs; reduce dosage prior to discontinuation.

GENERIC NAME	COMMON TRADE NAMES	THERAPEUTIC CATEGORY	PREPARATIONS	COMMON PEDIATRIC DOSAGE
Tobramycin Sulfate	NEBCIN	Antibacterial	Inj (per mL): 10, 40 mg Powd for Inj: 30 mg	Birth - 7 Days: Up to 4 mg/kg/day IM or IV in divided doses q 12 h. Over 7 Days: 6 - 7.5 mg/kg/day IM or IV in 3 or 4 equally divided doses.
Tolmetin Sodium	TOLECTIN 200 TOLECTIN DS TOLECTIN 600	Anti-Inflammatory	Tab: 200 mg Cpsl: 400 mg Tab: 600 mg	Juvenile Rheumatoid Arthritis (Over 2 yrs): 20 mg/kg/day po in divided doses (tid or qid).
Tolnaftate	AFTATE	Antifungal	Gel, Powder, Aerosol Powder & Liquid Spray: 1%	Apply a thin layer over affected area morning and night for 2 - 3 weeks.
	DESENEX		Spray Liquid: 1%	Apply to affected areas morning and night.
	DR. SCHOLL'S ATHLETE'S FOOT		Spray Powder & Spray Liquid: 1%	Apply liberally on entire infected area bid for for 2 weeks.
	TINACTIN		Cream, Solution, Powder, Aerosol Powder & Liquid Aerosol: 1%	Apply to affected areas morning and night for 2 - 3 weeks.
	TING		Cream, Powder, Aerosol Powder & Liquid Spray: 1%	Apply a thin layer over affected area morning and night for 2 - 4 weeks.
Triamcinolone	ARISTOCORT	Corticosteroid	Tab: 1, 2, 4, 8 mg	Initial dose may vary from 4 to 48 mg po per day. Dose requirements are variable and must be individualized based on the disease and the patient's response.

Triamcinolone Acetonide	ARISTOCORT A	Corticosteroid	**Cream:** 0.025, 0.1, 0.5% **Oint:** 0.1%	Apply to affected area as a thin film tid - qid depending on the severity of the condition.
	KENALOG		**Oint:** 0.025, 0.1, 0.5% **Cream:** 0.025, 0.1, 0.5%	Apply a thin film to the affected area bid - qid (of the 0.025%) or bid - tid (of the 0.1% or 0.5%). Rub in gently.
			Lotion: 0.025, 0.1%	Apply to the affected area bid - qid (of the 0.025%) or bid - tid (of the 0.1%). Rub in gently.
			Spray: 0.2%	Spray onto the affected area tid - qid.
	AZMACORT		**Aerosol:** 100 µg/spray	**6-12 yrs:** 1 - 2 inhalations (100 - 200 µg) tid or qid; or 2 - 4 inhalations (200 - 400 µg) bid. Maximum: 12 inhalations daily.
	KENALOG-40		**Inj:** 40 mg/mL	**6-12 yrs:** Suggested initial dose is 40 mg IM, although dosage depends more on the severity of symptoms than on age or weight.
Trifluoperazine Hydrochloride	STELAZINE	Antipsychotic	**Tab:** 1, 2, 5, 10 mg **Conc Liquid:** 10 mg/mL	**6-12 yrs:** 1 mg once daily or bid po.
			Inj: 2 mg/mL	**6-12 yrs:** 1 mg once daily or bid IM.
Triflupromazine Hydrochloride	VESPRIN	Antiemetic	**Inj:** 10, 20 mg/mL	**Over 2.5 yrs:** 0.2 - 0.25 mg/kg (0.1 - 0.125 mg/lb) IM. up to a maximum total dose of 10 mg/day.
Trifluridine	VIROPTIC	Antiviral	**Ophth Solution:** 1%	**Over 6 yrs:** 1 drop into affected eye(s) q 2 h while awake for a maximum of 9 drops daily until the cornea has re-epithelialized. Then use 1 drop q 4 h while awake for 7 days.
Trimethobenzamide Hydrochloride	TIGAN	Antiemetic	**Cpsl:** 100, 250 mg	**30-90 lbs:** 100 - 200 mg tid or qid po.
			Suppos: 100, 200 mg	**Under 30 lbs:** 100 mg tid or qid rectally. **30-90 lbs:** 100 - 200 mg tid or qid rectally.

GENERIC NAME	COMMON TRADE NAMES	THERAPEUTIC CATEGORY	PREPARATIONS	COMMON PEDIATRIC DOSAGE
Tripelennamine Hydrochloride	PBZ	Antihistamine	Tab: 25, 50 mg	**Except for Infants:** 5 mg/kg/day po divided into 4 - 6 doses. Maximum: 300 mg/day.
Trolamine Salicylate	MYOFLEX	Analgesic, Topical	Cream: 10%	**Over 2 yrs:** Apply to affected area not more than tid to qid.
Troleandomycin	TAO	Antibacterial	Cpsl: 250 mg	125 - 250 mg (3 - 5 mg/lb or 6.6 - 11 mg/kg) q 6 h po.
Tropicamide	MYDRIACYL	Mydriatic - Cycloplegic	Ophth Sol: 0.5, 1%	**Refraction:** 1 - 2 drops of the 1% solution into the eye(s). Repeat in 5 min. **Examination of Fundus:** 1 - 2 drops of the 0.5% solution into the eye(s), 15 - 20 min. prior to examination.
Tubocurarine Chloride		Neuromuscular Blocker	Inj: 3 mg (20 Units)/mL	**Induction and Maintenance in Neonates:** 0.3 mg/kg IV. **Older Children:** 0.6 mg/kg IV.
Urea	UREAPHIL	Osmotic Diuretic	Inj: 40 g/150 mL	After preparation of a 30% solution, inject 0.5 - 1.5 g/kg by slow IV infusion, at a rate not to exceed 4 mL/min. In children up to 2 years old, as little as 0.1 g/kg may be adequate.
Valproate Sodium	DEPACON	Antiepileptic	Inj: 100 mg/mL (valproic acid equivalent)	**Over 10 yrs:** Administer as a 60 minute IV infusion (≤ 20 mg/min) with the same frequency as the oral products (Divalproex sodium (DEPAKOTE) and Valproic acid (DEPAKENE)).
Valproic Acid	DEPAKENE	Antiepileptic	Syrup: 250 mg/5 mL Cpsl: 250 mg	Initially, 15 mg/kg/day po in 2 or 3 divided doses, increasing at 1 week intervals by 5 to 10 mg/kg/day. Maximum: 60 mg/kg/day.

Drug	Brand	Category	Forms	Dosage
Vancomycin Hydrochloride	VANCOCIN HCL	Antibacterial	Powd for Solution: 1, 10 g Cpsl: 125, 250 mg	**Pseudomembranous Colitis:** 40 mg/kg in 3 or 4 divided doses po for 7 - 10 days. Maximum: 2 g/day. **Neonates & Infants:** Initially, 15 mg/kg IV, followed by 10 mg/kg IV (given over 60 minutes) q 12 h for neonates in the 1st week of life and q 8 h thereafter up to 1 month of age. **Over 1 mo:** 10 mg/kg IV (given over 60 minutes) q 6 h.
Vecuronium Bromide	NORCURON	Neuromuscular Blocker	Powd for Inj: 10 mg	**7 wks - 1 yr:** These patients are moderately more sensitive to NORCURON on a mg/kg basis than adults and take about 1.5 times as long to recover. **1-10 yrs:** These patients may need a slightly higher initial dose and may need supplementation slightly more often than adults. **Over 10 yrs:** Initially 0.08 - 0.1 mg/kg as an IV bolus. Maintenance doses of 0.010 - 0.015 mg/kg are recommended and are usually required within 25 - 40 minutes after initial dose.
Verapamil Hydrochloride	ISOPTIN	Antiarrhythmic	Inj: 2.5 mg/mL	**Under 1 yr:** 0.1 - 0.2 mg/kg IV (as a bolus over at least 2 minutes) under continuous ECG monitoring. Repeat dose in 30 minutes if the response is not adequate. **1-15 yrs:** 0.1 - 0.3 mg/kg IV (as a bolus over at least 2 minutes). Do not exceed 5 mg. Repeat dose in 30 minutes if the response is not adequate. Do not exceed 10 mg as a single dose.
Vidarabine Monohydrate	VIRA-A	Antiviral	Ophth Oint: 3%	Apply 1/2 inch into the lower conjunctival sac 5 times daily at 3 hour intervals.

GENERIC NAME	COMMON TRADE NAMES	THERAPEUTIC CATEGORY	PREPARATIONS	COMMON PEDIATRIC DOSAGE
Vinblastine Sulfate	VELBAN	Antineoplastic	Powd for Inj: 10 mg	Dose at weekly intervals as follows: 1st dose — 2.5 mg/m^2 IV; 2nd dose — 3.75 mg/m^2 IV; 3rd dose — 5.0 mg/m^2 IV; 4th dose — 6.25 mg/m^2 IV; 5th dose — 7.5 mg/m^2 IV. The dose should not be increased after that dose which reduces the WBC to approximately 3,000 cells/mm^2.
Vincristine Sulfate	ONCOVIN	Antineoplastic	Inj: 1 mg/mL	**Usual Dose:** 2.0 mg/m^2 IV (at weekly intervals). **10 kg or less:** Starting dose should be 0.05 mg/kg IV (administered once weekly).
Vitamin A	AQUASOL A	Vitamin	Cpsl: 25,000 and 50,000 Units (7.5 and 15 mg of retinol, respectively)	**Over 8 yrs:** 100,000 Units daily po for 3 days followed by 50,000 units daily for 2 weeks. Follow-up therapy with an oral multivitamin preparation is recommended daily for 2 mos.
Vitamin A Palmitate	AQUASOL A	Vitamin	Inj: 50,000 Units (15 mg of retinol)/mL	**Infants:** 7,500 - 15,000 Units daily IM for 10 days. Follow-up therapy with an oral preparation (5,000 - 10,000 Units) is recommended for 2 mos. **1-8 yrs:** 17,500 - 35,000 Units daily IM for 10 days. Follow-up therapy with an oral preparation (5,000 - 10,000 Units) is recommended for 2 mos.
Xylometazoline Hydrochloride	CTRIVIN PEDIATRIC	Nasal Decongestant	Nasal Solution: 0.05%	**2-12 yrs:** 2 - 3 drops in each nostril q 8 - 10 h.
Zidovudine	RETROVIR	Antiviral	Syrup: 50 mg/5 mL Cpsl: 100 mg Tab: 300 mg	**Neonates:** 2 mg/kg po q 6 h starting within 12 h after birth and continuing through 6 weeks of age. **3 mos - 12 yrs:** 180 mg/m^2 q 6 h po (720 mg/m^2 daily), not to exceed 200 mg q 6 h.
			Inj: 10 mg/mL	**Neonates:** 1.5 mg/kg by IV infusion (over 30 min) q 6 h.

108

| Zinc Oxide | DESITIN CREAMY | Skin Protectant | Oint: 10% | Apply prn with each diaper change, especially hs. |
| | BALMEX | | Oint: 11.3% | At the first sign of diaper rash or redness, apply tid or more prn. To help prevent diaper rash, apply prn with each diaper change and hs. |

(C-II): Controlled Substance, Schedule II

(C-III): Controlled Substance, Schedule III

(C-IV): Controlled Substance, Schedule IV

Notes

SELECTED

COMBINATION

DRUG

PREPARATIONS

TRADE NAME	THERAPEUTIC CATEGORY	DOSAGE FORMS AND COMPOSITION	COMMON PEDIATRIC DOSAGE
A-200	Pediculicide	**Shampoo:** pyrethrum extract (0.33%), piperonyl butoxide (4%)	Apply to affected area until all the hair is thoroughly wet. Allow product to remain on the area for 10 minutes but no longer. Add sufficient warm water to form a lather and shampoo as usual. Rinse thoroughly. Remove dead lice and eggs from the hair with a fine-toothed comb. Repeat treatment in 7 - 10 days to kill any newly hatched lice.
A + D	Skin Protectant	**Oint:** petrolatum (53.4%), lanolin (15.5%)	Apply liberally prn with each diaper change, especially hs.
ACTIFED	Decongestant-Antihistamine	**Tab:** pseudoephedrine HCl (60 mg), triprolidine HCl (2.5 mg)	**6-12 yrs:** 1/2 tab q 4 - 6 h po.
ADDERALL 5 mg	CNS Stimulant	**Tab:** amphetamine asparate (1.25 mg), amphetamine sulfate (1.25 mg), dextroamphetamine saccharate (1.25 mg), dextroamphetamine sulfate (1.25 mg)	**Attention Deficit Disorder:** **3-5 yrs:** Start with 2.5 mg daily po. Daily dosage may be increased in increments of 2.5 mg at weekly intervals until the optimal response is obtained. **6 yrs and older:** Start with 5 mg once or twice daily po. Daily dosage may be increased in increments of 5 mg at weekly intervals until the optimal response is obtained. Give the 1st dose on awakening; additional doses (1 or 2) at intervals of 4 - 6 h.

112

ADDERALL 10 mg	CNS Stimulant	**Narcolepsy (6-12 yrs):** Initially, 5 mg daily po. Daily dosage may be increased in increments of 5 mg at weekly intervals until the optimal response is obtained. **Attention Deficit Disorder (6 yrs and older):** See dosage for ADDERALL 5 mg above. **Narcolepsy (6-12 yrs):** See dosage for ADDERALL 5 mg above.
	Tab: amphetamine asparate (2.5 mg), amphetamine sulfate (2.5 mg), dextroamphetamine saccharate (2.5 mg), dextroamphetamine sulfate (2.5 mg)	
AFRIN SALINE MIST	Nasal Moisturizer	2 - 6 sprays into each nostril prn.
	Nasal Spray: sodium chloride with sodium phosphate buffer	
AGORAL	Laxative	**6-12 yrs:** 2.5 - 3.75 mL po hs.
	Liquid Emulsion (per 15 mL): mineral oil (4.2 g), phenolphthalein (200 mg)	
ALDACTAZIDE	Diuretic	0.75 - 1.5 mg spironolactone/lb (1.65 - 3.3 mg/kg) daily po.
	Tab: spironolactone (25 mg), hydrochlorothiazide (25 mg) **Tab:** spironolactone (50 mg), hydrochlorothiazide (50 mg)	
ALKA-SELTZER GOLD	Antacid	1 tab fully dissolved in water q 4 h po, not to exceed 4 doses in 24 h.
	Effervescent Tab: sodium bicarbonate (958 mg), potassium bicarbonate (312 mg), citric acid (832 mg)	
ALKA-SELTZER PLUS COLD & COUGH MEDICINE	Analgesic-Antihistamine-Decongestant-Antitussive	**6-12 yrs:** 1 Liqui-Gel q 4 h po, not to exceed 4 doses in 24 h.
	Liqui-Gel: acetaminophen (325 mg), chlorpheniramine maleate (2 mg), pseudoephedrine HCl (30 mg), dextromethorphan HBr (10 mg)	
ALKA-SELTZER PLUS COLD & FLU (Non-Drowsy Formula)	Analgesic-Decongestant-Antitussive	**6-12 yrs:** 1 Liqui-Gel q 4 h po, not to exceed 4 doses in 24 h.
	Liqui-Gel: acetaminophen (325 mg), pseudoephedrine HCl (30 mg), dextromethorphan HBr (10 mg)	
ALKA-SELTZER PLUS COLD MEDICINE	Analgesic-Antihistamine-Decongestant	**6-12 yrs:** 1 Liqui-Gel q 4 h po, not to exceed 4 doses in 24 h.
	Liqui-Gel: acetaminophen (325 mg), chlorpheniramine maleate (2 mg), pseudoephedrine HCl (30 mg)	

TRADE NAME	THERAPEUTIC CATEGORY	DOSAGE FORMS AND COMPOSITION	COMMON PEDIATRIC DOSAGE
ALLEREST, CHILDREN'S	Decongestant-Antihistamine	**Chewable Tab:** phenylpropanolamine HCl (9.4 mg), chlorpheniramine maleate (1 mg)	**6-12 yrs:** 2 chewable tablets q 4 h po.
ALLEREST MAXIMUM STRENGTH	Decongestant-Antihistamine	**Tab:** pseudoephedrine HCl (30 mg), chlorpheniramine maleate (2 mg)	**6-12 yrs:** 1 tablet q 4 h po.
ALLEREST NO DROWSINESS	Analgesic-Decongestant	**Tab:** acetaminophen (325 mg), pseudoephedrine HCl (30 mg)	**6-12 yrs:** 1 tablet q 4 h po.
AMBENYL (C-V)	Antitussive-Antihistamine	**Syrup (per 5 mL):** codeine phosphate (10 mg), bromodiphenhydramine HCl (12.5 mg), alcohol (5%)	**6-12 yrs:** 2.5 - 5 mL q 6 h po.
ANACIN	Non-Opioid Analgesic, Antipyretic	**Tab & Cplt:** aspirin (400 mg), caffeine (32 mg)	**6-12 yrs:** 1 tablet or caplet q 4 h po.
ANALPRAM-HC 1%	Corticosteroid-Local Anesthetic	**Cream:** hydrocortisone acetate (1%), pramoxine HCl (1%)	Apply as a thin film to affected area tid - qid.
ANALPRAM-HC 2.5%	Corticosteroid-Local Anesthetic	**Cream & Lotion:** hydrocortisone acetate (2.5%), pramoxine HCl (1%)	Apply as a thin film to affected area tid - qid.
A.R.M.	Decongestant-Antihistamine	**Cplt:** phenylpropanolamine HCl (25 mg), chlorpheniramine maleate (4 mg)	**6-12 yrs:** 1/2 caplet q 4 h po.
ATROHIST PEDIATRIC	Decongestant-Antihistamine	**Susp (per 5 mL):** phenylephrine tannate (5 mg), chlorpheniramine tannate (2 mg), pyrilamine tannate (12.5 mg)	**2-6 yrs:** 2.5 - 5 mL q 12 h po. **6-12 yrs:** 5 - 10 mL q 12 h po.
AUGMENTIN 125	Antibacterial	**Powd for Susp (per 5 mL):** amoxicillin (125 mg), clavulanic acid (31.25 mg) **Chewable Tab:** amoxicillin (125 mg), clavulanic acid (31.25 mg)	All doses are based on the amoxicillin component. **Under 12 wks (3 mos):** 30 mg/kg/day divided q 12 h po. Use the 125 mg Suspension for this age group.

Drug	Category	Ingredients	Dosage
AUGMENTIN 200		**Powd for Susp (per 5 mL):** amoxicillin (200 mg), clavulanic acid (28.5 mg) **Chewable Tab:** amoxicillin (200 mg), clavulanic acid (28.5 mg)	**Over 3 mos:** **For Otitis Media, Sinusitis, Lower Respiratory, & More Severe Infections:** 45 mg/kg daily in divided doses q 12 h po or 40 mg/kg daily in divided doses q 8 h po. **Less Severe Infections:** 25 mg/kg daily in divided doses q 12 h po or 20 mg/kg daily in divided doses q 8 h po. **Children over 40 kg:** Use adult dosages, i.e., one 250 mg tab (AUGMENTIN 250) q 8 h po or one 500 mg tab (AUGMENTIN 500) q 12 h po.
AUGMENTIN 250		**Powd for Susp (per 5 mL):** amoxicillin (250 mg), clavulanic acid (62.5 mg) **Chewable Tab:** amoxicillin (250 mg), clavulanic acid (62.5 mg) **Tab:** amoxicillin (250 mg), clavulanic acid (125 mg)	
AUGMENTIN 400		**Powd for Susp (per 5 mL):** amoxicillin (400 mg), clavulanic acid (57 mg) **Chewable Tab:** amoxicillin (400 mg), clavulanic acid (57 mg)	
AUGMENTIN 500		**Tab:** amoxicillin (500 mg), clavulanic acid (125 mg)	
AURALGAN OTIC	Analgesic (Topical)	**Otic Solution (per mL):** benzocaine (14 mg = 1.4%), antipyrine (54 mg = 5.4%), glycerin	Instill in ear canal until filled, then insert a cotton pledget moistened with solution into meatus. Repeat q 1 - 2 h.
AVEENO ANTI-ITCH	Local Anesthetic-Skin Protectant	**Cream & Lotion:** pramoxine HCl (1.0%), camphor (0.3%), calamine (3.0%)	**Over 2 yrs:** Apply topically up to qid.
AYR	Nasal Moisturizer	**Nasal Solution & Spray:** sodium chloride (0.65%) with monobasic potassium phosphate/sodium hydroxide buffer	2 - 4 drops or 2 sprays into each nostril prn.
BACTINE ANTISEPTIC-ANESTHETIC	Antiseptic-Local Anesthetic	**Topical Liquid & Spray:** benzalkonium chloride (0.13%), lidocaine HCl (2.5%)	**Over 2 yrs:** Apply to affected areas 1 - 3 times daily.
BACTRIM	Antibacterial	**Tab:** trimethoprim (80 mg), sulfamethoxazole (400 mg) **Susp & Pediatric Susp (per 5 mL):** trimethoprim (40 mg), sulfamethoxazole (200 mg)	**Urinary Tract Infections or Acute Otitis Media (Over 2 mos):** 8 mg/kg trimethoprim and 40 mg/kg sulfamethoxazole po

TRADE NAME	THERAPEUTIC CATEGORY	DOSAGE FORMS AND COMPOSITION
BACTRIM DS		Tab: trimethoprim (160 mg), sulfamethoxazole (800 mg)

COMMON PEDIATRIC DOSAGE

per 24 h, given in 2 divided doses q 12 h for 10 days.
Dosage guideline (given q 12 h) based on child's weight -
10 kg or 22 lbs: 5 mL.
20 kg or 44 lbs: 10 mL. or 1 BACTRIM tablet.
30 kg or 66 lbs: 15 mL. or 1.5 BACTRIM tablets.
40 kg or 88 lbs: 20 mL, 2 BACTRIM tablets, or 1 BACTRIM DS tablet.
Shigellosis (Over 2 mos): Same daily dose is used for 5 days po.

Pneumocystis carinii **Pneumonia**
Treatment (Over 2 mos):
15 - 20 mg/kg trimethoprim and 75 - 100 mg/kg sulfamethoxazole po per 24 h in equally divided doses q 6 h for 14 - 21 days.
Dosage guideline (given q 6 h) based on child's weight -
8 kg or 18 lbs: 5 mL.
16 kg or 35 lbs: 10 mL. or 1 BACTRIM tablet.
24 kg or 53 lbs: 15 mL. or 1.5 BACTRIM tablets.
32 kg or 70 lbs: 20 mL, 2 BACTRIM tablets, or 1 BACTRIM DS tablet.

116

			***Pneumocystis carinii* Pneumonia Prophylaxis (Over 2 mos):** 150 mg/m^2 trimethoprim and 750 mg/m^2 sulfamethoxazole po per 24 h in equally divided doses bid on 3 consecutive days per week. The total daily dose should not exceed 320 mg trimethoprim and 1600 mg sulfamethoxazole. Dosage guideline based on child's body surface area - **0.26 m^2**: 2.5 mL. **0.53 m^2**: 5 mL or 1/2 BACTRIM tablet. **1.06 m^2**: 10 mL or 1 BACTRIM tablet.
BACTRIM I.V. INFUSION	Antibacterial	**Inj (per 5 mL)**: trimethoprim (80 mg), sulfamethoxazole (400 mg)	**Severe Urinary Tract Infections and Shigellosis (Over 2 mos):** 8 - 10 mg/kg daily (based on trimethoprim) in 2 - 4 equally divided doses q 6, 8 or 12 h by IV infusion for up to 14 days for UTI and 5 days for shigellosis. ***Pneumocystis carinii* Pneumonia (Over 2 mos):** 15 - 20 mg/kg daily (based on trimethoprim) in 3 - 4 equally divided doses q 6 - 8 h by IV infusion for up to 14 days.
BENADRYL ALLERGY / CONGESTION	Decongestant-Antihistamine	**Liquid (per 5 mL)**: pseudoephedrine HCl (30 mg), diphenhydramine HCl (12.5 mg)	**6-12 yrs:** 5 mL q 4 - 6 h po, not to exceed 20 mL in 24 h.
BENADRYL ITCH RELIEF	Antihistamine-Skin Protectant	**Stick**: diphenhydramine HCl (2%), zinc acetate (0.1%, alcohol (73.5%)	**6-12 yrs:** Apply to the affected area not more than tid or qid.

TRADE NAME	THERAPEUTIC CATEGORY	DOSAGE FORMS AND COMPOSITION	COMMON PEDIATRIC DOSAGE
BENADRYL ITCH STOPPING CREAM & SPRAY - Original Strength	Antihistamine-Skin Protectant	Cream & Spray: diphenhydramine (1%), zinc acetate (0.1%)	2-12 yrs: Apply to affected areas not more than tid to qid.
BENYLIN EXPECTORANT	Antitussive-Expectorant	Liquid (per 5 mL): dextromethorphan HBr (5 mg), guaifenesin (100 mg)	2-6 yrs (24-47 lbs): 2.5 - 5 mL q 4 h po. 6-12 yrs (48-95 lbs): 5 - 10 mL q 4 h po.
BENYLIN MULTISYMPTOM	Antitussive-Expectorant-Decongestant	Liquid (per 5 mL): dextromethorphan HBr (5 mg), guaifenesin (100 mg), pseudoephedrine HCl (15 mg)	2-6 yrs: 5 mL q 4 h po, not to exceed 4 doses in 24 h. 6-12 yrs: 10 mL q 4 h po, not to exceed 4 doses in 24 h.
BICILLIN C-R	Antibacterial	Inj (per mL): penicillin G benzathine (150,000 Units), penicillin G procaine (150,000 Units) Inj (per mL): penicillin G benzathine (300,000 Units), penicillin G procaine (300,000 Units)	Streptococcal Infections: Under 30 lbs: 600,000 Units daily by deep IM injection (at multiple sites). 30-60 lbs: 900,000 to 1,200,000 Units daily by deep IM injection (at multiple sites). Over 60 lbs: 2,400,000 Units daily by deep IM injection (at multiple sites). Pneumococcal Infections (except Meningitis): 600,000 Units q 2 - 3 days by deep IM injection until the body temp. is normal for 48 h.

BICILLIN C-R 900/300	Antibacterial	**Inj (per 2 mL):** penicillin G benzathine (900,000 Units), penicillin G procaine (300,000 units)	**Streptococcal Infections:** A single deep IM injection is usually sufficient. **Pneumococcal Infections (except Meningitis):** One 2 mL deep IM injection, repeated q 2 - 3 days until the body temp. is normal for 48 hours.
BLEPHAMIDE	Antibacterial-Corticosteroid	**Ophth Susp:** sulfacetamide sodium (10%), prednisolone acetate (0.2%)	**Over 6 yrs:** 1 drop into the affected eye(s) bid - qid, depending on the severity of the condition.
		Ophth Oint: sulfacetamide sodium (10%), prednisolone acetate (0.2%)	**Over 6 yrs:** Apply approx. 1/2 in to the conjunctival sac tid to qid and once or twice at night.
BOROFAX	Diaper Rash Product	**Oint:** zinc oxide (15%), white petrolatum (68.6%)	After cleaning the diaper area and drying, apply liberally prn with each diaper change.
BROMFED	Decongestant-Antihistamine	**Tab:** pseudoephedrine HCl (60 mg), brompheniramine maleate (4 mg)	**Over 6 yrs:** 1/2 tab q 4 h po.
BROMFED-DM	Decongestant-Antihistamine-Antitussive	**Syrup (per 5 mL):** pseudoephedrine HCl (30 mg), brompheniramine maleate (2 mg), dextromethorphan HBr (10 mg)	**2-6 yrs:** 2.5 mL q 4 h po. **6-12 yrs:** 5 mL q 4 h po.
BROMFED-PD	Decongestant-Antihistamine	**Extended-Rel. Cpsl:** pseudoephedrine HCl (60 mg), brompheniramine maleate (6 mg)	**6-12 yrs:** 1 cpsl q 12 h po.
BRONTEX LIQUID (C-V)	Antitussive-Expectorant	**Liquid (per 10 mL):** codeine phosphate (5 mg), guaifenesin (150 mg)	**6-12 yrs:** 10 mL q 4 h po, prn.
BUFFERIN	Analgesic, Antipyretic	**Cplt & Tab:** aspirin (325 mg), calcium carbonate (158 mg), magnesium oxide (63 mg), magnesium carbonate (34 mg)	**6-12 yrs:** 1 caplet (or tablet) q 4 h po, prn. Do not exceed 5 caplets (or tablets) in 24 h.

119

TRADE NAME	THERAPEUTIC CATEGORY	DOSAGE FORMS AND COMPOSITION	COMMON PEDIATRIC DOSAGE
CALADRYL	Antihistamine-Skin Protectant	Cream & Lotion: pramoxine HCl (1%), calamine (8%) Clear Lotion: pramoxine HCl (1%), zinc acetate (0.1%)	Over 2 yrs: Apply to affected area(s) tid to qid.
CALDESENE	Diaper Rash Product	Oint: zinc oxide (15%), white petrolatum (53.9%)	After cleaning the diaper area and drying, apply liberally prn with each diaper change.
CAMPHO-PHENIQUE ANTISEPTIC	Topical Analgesic	Gel & Liquid: camphorated phenol (camphor (10.8%), phenol (4.7%) in light mineral oil)	Clean the affected area. Apply with cotton 1 - 3 times daily.
CAMPHO-PHENIQUE FIRST AID ANTIBIOTIC PLUS PAIN RELIEVER	Antibacterial-Local Anesthetic	Oint (per g): polymyxin B sulfate (10,000 Units), neomycin sulfate (equal to 3.5 mg of neomycin base), bacitracin zinc (500 Units), lidocaine HCl (40 mg)	Over 2 yrs: Apply topically 1 - 3 times daily to affected areas.
CEPACOL SORE THROAT FORMULA, CHILDREN'S	Decongestant-Analgesic	Liquid (per 5 mL): pseudoephedrine HCl (15 mg), acetaminophen (160 mg)	2-5 yrs (24-47 lbs): 5 mL q 4 to 6 h po, not to exceed 4 doses in 24 h. 6-11 yrs (48-95 lbs): 10 mL q 4 to 6 h po, not to exceed 4 doses in 24 h. 12 yrs and over (over 95 lbs): 20 mL q 4 - 6 h po, not to exceed 4 doses in 24 h.
CEPACOL SORE THROAT LOZENGES (Maximum Strength)	Local Anesthetic (Oral)	Lozenge (Mint): benzocaine (10 mg), menthol (2 mg) Lozenge (Cool Mint): benzocaine (10 mg), menthol (2.5 mg) Lozenge (Cherry): benzocaine (10 mg), menthol (3.6 mg) Lozenge (Sugar-Free Cherry): benzocaine (10 mg), menthol (4.5 mg)	Over 6 yrs: Dissolve 1 in the mouth q 2 h prn.
CEROSE-DM	Decongestant-Antihistamine-Antitussive	Liquid (per 5 mL): phenylephrine HCl (10 mg), chlorpheniramine maleate (4 mg), dextromethorphan HBr (15 mg), alcohol (2.4%)	6-12 yrs: 2.5 mL qid po prn.
CETAPRED	Antibacterial-Corticosteroid	Ophth Oint: sulfacetamide sodium (10%), prednisolone acetate (0.25%)	Over 6 yrs: Apply a small amount to the affected eye(s) tid to qid and once or twice at night.

120

CETAPRED, ISOPTO	Antibacterial-Corticosteroid	**Ophth Susp:** sulfacetamide sodium (10%), prednisolone acetate (0.25%)	**Over 6 yrs:** 2 drops into the affected eye(s) q 4 h.
CHERACOL (C-V)	Antitussive-Expectorant	**Syrup (per 5 mL):** codeine phosphate (10 mg), guaifenesin (100 mg), alcohol (4.75%)	**6-12 yrs:** 5 mL q 4 - 6 h po.
CHERACOL-D	Antitussive-Expectorant	**Liquid (per 5 mL):** dextromethorphan HBr (10 mg), guaifenesin (100 mg), alcohol (4.75%)	**2-6 yrs:** 2.5 mL q 4 h po. **6-12 yrs:** 5 mL q 4 h po.
CHLORASEPTIC SORE THROAT LOZENGES	Local Anesthetic (Oral)	**Lozenge:** benzocaine (6 mg), menthol (10 mg)	**Over 5 yrs:** Dissolve 1 slowly in the mouth. May repeat q 2 h prn.
CHLOROMYCETIN HYDROCORTISONE	Antibacterial-Corticosteroid	**Powd for Ophth Susp:** chloramphenicol (12.5 mg), hydrocortisone acetate (25 mg) in vials with diluent	2 drops in the affected eye(s) q 3 h. Continue dosing day & night for the first 48 h, after which the interval between applications may be increased. Treatment should continue for 48 h after the eye appears normal.
CHLOR-TRIMETON 4 HOUR ALLERGY/ DECONGESTANT	Decongestant-Antihistamine	**Tab:** pseudoephedrine (60 mg), chlorpheniramine maleate (4 mg)	**6-12 yrs:** 1/2 tab q 4 - 6 h po.
CODICLEAR DH (C-III)	Antitussive-Expectorant	**Syrup (per 5 mL):** hydrocodone bitartrate (5 mg), guaifenesin (100 mg)	**6-12 yrs:** 2.5 mL po pc & hs, not less than 4 h apart.
CODIMAL DH (C-III)	Decongestant-Antihistamine-Antitussive	**Syrup (per 5 mL):** phenylephrine HCl (5 mg), pyrilamine maleate (8.33 mg), hydrocodone bitartrate (1.66 mg)	**2-6 yrs:** 2.5 mL q 4 h po. **6-12 yrs:** 5 mL q 4 h po.
CODIMAL-L.A. HALF CAPSULES	Decongestant-Antihistamine	**Cpsl:** pseudoephedrine HCl (60 mg), chlorpheniramine maleate (4 mg)	**6-12 yrs:** 1 cpsl q 12 h po.
COLY-MYCIN S OTIC	Antibacterial-Corticosteroid	**Otic Susp (per mL):** neomycin sulfate (4.71 mg, equivalent to 3.3 mg neomycin base), colistin sulfate (3 mg), hydrocortisone acetate (10 mg = 1%)	4 drops instilled into the affected ear(s) tid - qid.
CONGESTAC	Decongestant-Expectorant	**Cplt:** pseudoephedrine HCl (60 mg), guaifenesin (400 mg)	**6-12 yrs:** 1/2 caplet q 4 h po.

TRADE NAME	THERAPEUTIC CATEGORY	DOSAGE FORMS AND COMPOSITION	COMMON PEDIATRIC DOSAGE
CORICIDIN HBP COLD & FLU	Analgesic-Antihistamine	**Tab:** acetaminophen (325 mg), chlorpheniramine maleate (2 mg)	**6-12 yrs:** 1 tab q 4 - 6 h po, not to exceed 5 tablets in 24 h.
CORICIDIN HBP NIGHT-TIME COLD & COUGH	Analgesic-Antihistamine	**Liquid (per 15 mL):** acetaminophen (325 mg), diphenhydramine HCl (12.5 mg)	**6-12 yrs:** 15 mL q 4 h po, not to exceed 5 doses in 24 h.
CORICIDIN "D"	Analgesic-Antihistamine-Decongestant	**Tab:** acetaminophen (325 mg), chlorpheniramine maleate (2 mg), phenylpropanolamine HCl (12.5 mg)	**6-11 yrs:** 1 tab q 4 h po, not to exceed 5 tablets in 24 h.
CORTISPORIN	Antibacterial-Corticosteroid	**Ophth Susp (per mL):** polymyxin B sulfate (10,000 Units), neomycin sulfate (equal to 3.5 mg of neomycin base), hydrocortisone (10 mg = 1%)	1 - 2 drops into the affected eye(s) q 3 - 4 h, depending on the severity of the condition.
		Ophth Oint (per g): polymyxin B sulfate (10,000 Units), neomycin sulfate (equal to 3.5 mg of neomycin base), bacitracin zinc (400 Units), hydrocortisone (10 mg = 1%)	Apply to the affected eye(s) q 3 - 4 h, depending on the severity of the condition.
		Otic Solution & Susp (per mL): polymyxin B sulfate (10,000 Units), neomycin sulfate (equal to 3.5 mg of neomycin base), hydrocortisone (10 mg = 1%)	3 drops instilled in the affected ear(s) tid to qid.
		Cream (per g): polymyxin B sulfate (10,000 Units), neomycin sulfate (equal to 3.5 mg of neomycin base), hydrocortisone acetate (5 mg = 0.5%)	Apply topically bid - qid. If the conditions permit, gently rub into the affected areas.
		Oint (per g): polymyxin B sulfate (5,000 Units), neomycin sulfate (equal to 3.5 mg of neomycin base), bacitracin zinc (400 Units), hydrocortisone (10 mg = 1%)	Apply topically as a thin film bid to qid prn.
COUGH-X	Antitussive-Local Anesthetic (Oral)	**Lozenge:** dextromethorphan HBr (5 mg), benzocaine (2 mg)	**2-6 yrs:** Dissolve 1 lozenge in the mouth q 4 h. **6-12 yrs:** Dissolve 1 lozenge in the mouth q 2 h.
CRUEX (Original)	Antifungal	**Spray Powder:** total undecylenate = 19% as undecylenic acid and zinc undecylenate	**Over 2 yrs:** Spray a thin layer onto the affected skin areas bid, AM and PM.

122

D.A. II	Decongestant-Antihistamine-Anticholinergic	**Long-Acting Tab:** phenylephrine HCl (10 mg), chlorpheniramine maleate (4 mg), methscopolamine nitrate (1.25 mg)	**6-12 yrs:** 1 tab q 12 h po.
DECONAMINE	Decongestant-Antihistamine	**Syrup (per 5 mL):** pseudoephedrine HCl (30 mg), chlorpheniramine maleate (2 mg)	**2-6 yrs:** 2.5 mL tid or qid po. **6-12 yrs:** 2.5 - 5 mL tid or qid po.
DECONSAL II	Decongestant-Expectorant	**Extended-Rel. Tab:** pseudoephedrine HCl (60 mg), guaifenesin (600 mg)	**2-6 yrs:** 1/2 tab q 12 h po. **6-12 yrs:** 1 tab q 12 h po.
DESENEX (Original)	Antifungal	**Oint, Powder, & Spray Powder:** total undecylenate = 25% as undecylenic acid and zinc undecylenate	**Over 2 yrs:** Apply a thin layer to the affected skin areas bid, AM and PM.
DESITIN	Skin Protectant	**Oint:** zinc oxide (40%), cod liver oil	**Prevention of Diaper Rash:** Apply to the diaper area, especially hs. **Treatment of Diaper Rash:** Apply to affected area tid - qid prn.
DEXACIDIN	Antibacterial-Corticosteroid	**Ophth Oint (per g):** neomycin sulfate (equal to 3.5 mg of neomycin base), polymyxin B sulfate (10,000 Units), dexamethasone (1 mg)	Apply a small amount (about 0.5 in.) into the conjunctival sac tid - qid.
DIALOSE PLUS	Stimulant Laxative-Stool Softener	**Tab:** yellow phenolphthalein (65 mg), docusate sodium (100 mg)	**6-12 yrs:** 1 tablet daily po.
DICAL-D	Calcium Supplement	**Tab:** dibasic calcium phosphate (500 mg), cholecalciferol (3.33 µg)	**Over 4 yrs:** 1 tab tid po with meals.
DIMACOL	Antitussive-Decongestant-Expectorant	**Cplt:** dextromethorphan HBr (10 mg), pseudoephedrine HCl (30 mg), guaifenesin (100 mg)	**6-12 yrs:** 1 caplet q 4 h po.
DIMETANE DECONGESTANT	Decongestant-Antihistamine	**Elixir (per 5 mL):** phenylephrine HCl (5 mg), brompheniramine maleate (2 mg), alcohol (2.3%) **Cplt:** phenylephrine HCl (10 mg), brompheniramine maleate (4 mg)	**6-12 yrs:** 5 mL q 4 h po. **6-12 yrs:** 1/2 caplet q 4 h po.

TRADE NAME	THERAPEUTIC CATEGORY	DOSAGE FORMS AND COMPOSITION	COMMON PEDIATRIC DOSAGE
DIMETANE-DC (C-V)	Antitussive-Decongestant-Antihistamine	Syrup (per 5 ml): codeine phosphate (10 mg), phenylpropanolamine HCl (12.5 mg), brompheniramine maleate (2 mg), alcohol (0.95%)	2-6 yrs: 2.5 mL q 4 h po. 6-12 yrs: 5 mL q 4 h po.
DIMETANE-DX	Antitussive-Decongestant-Antihistamine	Syrup (per 5 mL): dextromethorphan HBr (10 mg), pseudoephedrine HCl (30 mg), brompheniramine maleate (2 mg), alcohol (0.95%)	2-6 yrs: 2.5 mL q 4 h po. 6-12 yrs: 5 mL q 4 h po.
DIMETAPP	Decongestant-Antihistamine	Elixir (per 5 mL): phenylpropanolamine HCl (12.5 mg), brompheniramine maleate (2 mg)	6-12 yrs: 5 mL q 4 h po.
		Tab: phenylpropanolamine HCl (25 mg), brompheniramine maleate (4 mg)	6-12 yrs: 1/2 tablet q 4 h po.
DIMETAPP COLD & ALLERGY	Decongestant-Antihistamine	Chewable Tab: phenylpropanolamine HCl (6.25 mg), brompheniramine maleate (1 mg)	2-6 yrs: 1 tab q 4 h po. 6-12 yrs: 2 tabs q 4 h po.
DIMETAPP COLD AND FEVER	Decongestant-Antihistamine-Analgesic	Susp (per 5 mL): pseudoephedrine HCl (15 mg), brompheniramine maleate (1 mg), acetaminophen (160 mg)	6-12 yrs: 10 mL q 4 h po. Do not exceed 4 doses in 24 h.
DIMETAPP DM	Decongestant-Antihistamine-Antitussive	Elixir (per 5 mL): phenylpropanolamine HCl (12.5 mg), brompheniramine maleate (2 mg), dextromethorphan HBr (10 mg)	6-12 yrs: 5 mL q 4 h po.
DOMEBORO	Astringent	Powder (per packet): aluminum sulfate (1191 mg), calcium acetate (938 mg) Effervescent Tab: aluminum sulfate (878 mg), calcium acetate (604 mg)	As a Compress: Dissolve 1 or 2 packets (or tabs) in 16 fl. oz. of warm water. Saturate a clean dressing in the sol'n, gently squeeze and apply loosely to the affected area. Remove, remoisten and reapply q 15 - 30 minutes prn. As a Soak: Dissolve 1 or 2 packets (or tabs) in 16 fl. oz. of warm water. Soak the affected area for 15 - 30 minutes. Repeat tid.

DONNATAL	Antispasmodic, Anticholinergic	**Elixir (per 5 mL):** atropine sulfate (0.0194 mg), scopolamine HBr (0.0065 mg), hyoscyamine sulfate (0.1037 mg), phenobarbital (16.2 mg), alcohol (23%)	0.5 mL/10 lbs q 4 h po or 0.75 mL/10 lbs q 6 h po.
DORCOL CHILDREN'S COUGH SYRUP	Decongestant-Expectorant-Antitussive	**Syrup (per 5 mL):** pseudoephedrine HCl (15 mg), guaifenesin (50 mg), dextromethorphan HBr (5 mg)	**3-12 mos:** 3 drops/kg q 4 h po. **1-2 yrs:** 7 drops (0.2 mL)/kg q 4 h po. **2-6 yrs (25-45 lbs):** 5 mL q 4 h po. **6-12 yrs (46-85 lbs):** 10 mL q 4 h po.
DORCOL CHILDREN'S LIQUID COLD FORMULA	Decongestant-Antihistamine	**Liquid (per 5 mL):** pseudoephedrine HCl (15 mg), chlorpheniramine maleate (1 mg)	**3-12 mos:** 2 drops/kg q 4 - 6 h po. **1-2 yrs:** 5 drops (0.2 mL)/kg q 4 - 6 h po. **2-6 yrs (25-45 lbs):** 5 mL q 4 - 6 h po. **6-12 yrs (46-85 lbs):** 10 mL q 4 - 6 h po.
DOXIDAN	Stimulant Laxative-Stool Softener	**Liqui-Gel:** casanthranol (30 mg), docusate sodium (100 mg)	**2-12 yrs:** 1 Liqui-Gel daily po.
DRISTAN COLD	Decongestant-Antihistamine-Analgesic	**Tab:** phenylephrine HCl (5 mg), chlorpheniramine maleate (2 mg), acetaminophen (325 mg)	**6-12 yrs:** 1 tablet q 4 h po.
DRIXORAL	Decongestant-Antihistamine	**Syrup (per 5 mL):** pseudoephedrine sulfate (30 mg), brompheniramine maleate (2 mg)	**6-12 yrs:** 5 mL q 4 - 6 h po.
DURATUSS	Decongestant-Expectorant	**Sustained-Rel. Tab:** pseudoephedrine HCl (120 mg), guaifenesin (600 mg)	**6-12 yrs:** 1/2 tab q 12 h po.
DURATUSS DM	Antitussive-Expectorant	**Elixir (per 5 mL):** dextromethorphan HBr (20 mg), guaifenesin (200 mg), alcohol (5%)	**2-6 yrs:** 1.25 mL q 4 h po. **6-12 yrs:** 2.5 mL q 4 h po.
DURATUSS HD (C-III)	Antitussive-Decongestant-Expectorant	**Elixir (per 5 mL):** hydrocodone bitartrate (2.5 mg), pseudoephedrine HCl (30 mg), guaifenesin (100 mg), alcohol (5%)	**6-12 yrs:** 5 mL q 4 - 6 h po.

125

TRADE NAME	THERAPEUTIC CATEGORY	DOSAGE FORMS AND COMPOSITION	COMMON PEDIATRIC DOSAGE
DURA-VENT	Decongestant-Expectorant	**Long-Acting Tab**: phenylpropanolamine HCl (75 mg), guaifensin (600 mg)	**6-12 yrs**: 1/2 tab q 12 h po.
DURA-VENT/DA	Decongestant-Antihistamine-Anticholinergic	**Long-Acting Tab**: phenylephrine HCl (20 mg), chlorpheniramine maleate (8 mg), methscopolamine nitrate (2.5 mg)	**6-12 yrs**: 1/2 tab q 12 h po.
ELIXOPHYLLIN-GG	Antiasthmatic	**Liquid (per 15 mL)**: theophylline anhydrous (100 mg), guaifenesin (100 mg)	Dose based on theophylline; see the Theophylline Table, Section I., p. 158.
EMETROL	Antiemetic	**Solution (per 5 mL)**: dextrose (1.87 g), levulose (1.87 g), phosphoric acid (21.5 mg)	5 - 10 mL po. Repeat q 15 minutes until the distress subsides.
ENTEX	Decongestant-Expectorant	**Liquid (per 5 mL)**: phenylephrine HCl (5 mg), phenylpropanolamine HCl (20 mg), guaifenesin (100 mg), alcohol (5%)	**2-4 yrs**: 2.5 mL qid po. **4-6 yrs**: 5 mL qid po. **6-12 yrs**: 7.5 mL qid po.
ENTEX LA	Decongestant-Expectorant	**Long-Acting Tab**: phenylpropanolamine HCl (75 mg), guaifenesin (400 mg)	**6-12 yrs**: 1/2 tab bid (q 12 h) po.
ENTEX PSE	Decongestant-Expectorant	**Long-Acting Tab**: pseudoephedrine HCl (120 mg), guaifenesin (600 mg)	**6-12 yrs**: 1/2 tab bid (q 12 h) po.
EXGEST LA	Decongestant-Expectorant	**Long-Acting Tab**: phenylpropanolamine HCl (75 mg), guaifenesin (400 mg)	**6-12 yrs**: 1/2 tab q 12 h po.
EXTENDRYL	Decongestant-Antihistamine-Anticholinergic	**Syrup (per 5 mL)**: phenylephrine HCl (10 mg), chlorpheniramine maleate (2 mg), methscopolamine nitrate (1.25 mg) **Tab**: phenylephrine HCl (10 mg), chlorpheniramine maleate (2 mg), methscopolamine nitrate (1.25 mg)	**6-12 yrs**: 5 mL q 4 h po. **6-12 yrs**: 1 tab q 4 h po.
EXTENDRYL JR	Decongestant-Antihistamine-Anticholinergic	**Sustained-Release Cpsl**: phenylephrine HCl (10 mg), chlorpheniramine maleate (4 mg), methscopolamine nitrate (1.25 mg)	**6-12 yrs**: 1 cpsl q 12 h po.

FANSIDAR	Antimalarial	Tab: sulfadoxine (500 mg), pyrimethamine (25 mg)	**Acute Malarial Attack:** Under 4 yrs: 1/2 tab po. 4-8 yrs: 1 tab po. 9-14 yrs: 2 tab po. **Malaria Prophylaxis:** Under 4 yrs: 1/4 tab po once weekly or 1/2 tab q 2 wks. 4-8 yrs: 1/2 tab po once weekly or 1 tab q 2 wks. 9-14 yrs: 3/4 tab po once weekly or 1.5 tab q 2 wks. Begin 1 - 2 days before departure to an endemic area; continue during stay and for 4 to 6 weeks after return.
FEDAHIST EXPECTORANT	Decongestant-Expectorant	Syrup (per 5 mL): pseudoephedrine HCl (20 mg), guaifenesin (200 mg).	2-5 yrs: 2.5 mL q 4 - 6 h po. 6-12 yrs: 5 mL q 4 - 6 h po.
FERANCEE	Hematinic	Chewable Tab: ferrous fumarate (200 mg), vitamin C (150 mg from ascorbic acid and sodium ascorbate)	6-12 yrs: 1 tablet daily po.
FLEET ENEMA FOR CHILDREN	Saline Laxative	Rectal Solution (per 59 mL): monobasic sodium phosphate (9.5 g), dibasic sodium phosphate (3.5 g)	2-12 yrs: Administer entire 2 fl. oz. rectally as a single dose.
FLEET PHOSPHO-SODA	Saline Laxative	Solution (per 5 mL): monobasic sodium phosphate (2.4 g), dibasic sodium phosphate (0.9 g)	5-10 yrs: 5 mL po as a single daily dose. 10-12 yrs: 10 mL po as a single daily dose.
4-WAY COLD	Decongestant-Antihistamine-Analgesic	Tab: phenylpropanolamine HCl (12.5 mg), chlorpheniramine maleate (2 mg), acetaminophen (325 mg)	6-12 yrs: 1 tablet q 4 h po, not to exceed 5 tablets in 24 h.
GUAIFED	Decongestant-Expectorant	Syrup (per 5 mL): pseudoephedrine HCl (30 mg), guaifenesin (200 mg)	2-6 yrs: 2.5 mL q 4 - 6 h po, not to exceed 10 mL in 24 h. 6-12 yrs: 5 mL q 4 - 6 h po, not to exceed 20 mL in 24 h.
GUAIFED-PD	Decongestant-Expectorant	Cpsl: pseudoephedrine HCl (60 mg), guaifenesin (300 mg)	6-12 yrs: 1 cpsl q 12 h po.

127

TRADE NAME	THERAPEUTIC CATEGORY	DOSAGE FORMS AND COMPOSITION	COMMON PEDIATRIC DOSAGE
GUAIMAX-D	Decongestant-Expectorant	**Extended-Rel. Tab:** pseudoephedrine HCl (120 mg), guaifenesin (600 mg)	**6-12 yrs:** 1/2 tab q 12 h po.
GUAITAB	Decongestant-Expectorant	**Tab:** pseudoephedrine HCl (60 mg), guaifenesin (400 mg)	**6-12 yrs:** 1/2 tablet q 4 - 6 h po, not to exceed 2 tablets in 24 h.
HALEY'S M-O	Laxative	**Liquid (per 5 mL):** mineral oil (1.25 mL), magnesium hydroxide (304 mg)	**6-12 yrs:** 5 mL daily po.
HYCODAN (C-III)	Antitussive-Anticholinergic	**Syrup (per 5 mL):** hydrocodone bitartrate (5 mg), homatropine methylbromide (1.5 mg)	**6-12 yrs:** 2.5 mL q 4 - 6 h po.
		Tab: hydrocodone bitartrate (5 mg), homatropine methylbromide (1.5 mg)	**6-12 yrs:** 1/2 tab q 4 - 6 h po.
HYCOMINE COMPOUND (C-III)	Antitussive-Decongestant-Antihistamine-Analgesic	**Tab:** hydrocodone bitartrate (5 mg), phenylephrine HCl (10 mg), chlorpheniramine maleate (2 mg), acetaminophen (250 mg), caffeine (30 mg)	**6-12 yrs:** 1/2 tab qid po.
HYCOMINE PEDIATRIC (C-III)	Antitussive-Decongestant	**Syrup (per 5 mL):** hydrocodone bitartrate (2.5 mg), phenylpropanolamine HCl (12.5 mg)	**6-12 yrs:** 5 mL q 4 h po.
HYCOTUSS EXPECTORANT (C-III)	Antitussive-Expectorant	**Syrup (per 5 mL):** hydrocodone bitartrate (5 mg), guaifenesin (100 mg), alcohol (10%)	**6-12 yrs:** 2.5 mL q 4 h po.
IMODIUM ADVANCED	Antidiarrheal-Antiflatulant	**Chewable Tab:** loperamide HCl (2 mg), simethicone (125 mg)	**6-8 yrs (48-59 lbs):** Chew 1 tab after the first loose bowel movement, then 1/2 tab after each subsequent loose bowel movement. Maximum: 2 tabs daily for 2 days. **9-11 yrs (60-95 lbs):** Chew 1 tab after the first loose bowel movement, then 1/2 tab after each subsequent loose bowel movement. Maximum: 3 tabs daily for 2 days.

Iodine	Antiseptic	**Solution & Tincture:** iodine (2%), sodium iodide (2.4%)	Apply to affected areas up to tid.
ITCH-X	Local Anesthetic (Topical)	**Gel:** pramoxine HCl (1%), benzyl alcohol (10%)	**Over 2 yrs:** Apply to affected areas not more than tid or qid.
KRONOFED-A-JR	Decongestant-Antihistamine	**Sustained-Rel. Cpsl:** pseudoephedrine HCl (60 mg), chlorpheniramine maleate (4 mg)	**6-12 yrs:** 1 cpsl q 12 h po.
LOMOTIL (C-V)	Antidiarrheal	**Liquid (per 5 mL):** diphenoxylate HCl (2.5 mg), atropine sulfate (0.025 mg), alcohol (15%)	**Over 2 yrs:** 0.3 - 0.4 mg/kg po in 4 divided doses, or by age or weight - **2 yrs (24-31 lbs):** 1.5 - 3.0 mL qid po. **3 yrs (26-35 lbs):** 2.0 - 3.0 mL qid po. **4 yrs (31-44 lbs):** 2.0 - 4.0 mL qid po. **5 yrs (35-51 lbs):** 2.5 - 4.5 mL qid po. **6-8 yrs (38-71 lbs):** 2.5 - 5.0 mL qid po. **9-12 yrs (51-121 lbs):** 3.5 to 5.0 mL qid po.
LUFYLLIN-GG	Antiasthmatic	**Elixir (per 15 mL):** dyphylline (100 mg), guaifenesin (100 mg), alcohol (17%) **Tab:** dyphylline (200 mg), guaifenesin (200 mg)	**Over 6 yrs:** 15 - 30 mL tid or qid po. **Over 6 yrs:** 1/2 - 1 tab tid or qid po.
MARAX	Antiasthmatic	**Tab:** theophylline (130 mg), ephedrine sulfate (25 mg), hydroxyzine HCl (10 mg)	**Over 5 yrs:** 1/2 tab bid - qid po. Some patients are adequately controlled with 1/4 - 1/2 tab hs.
MARAX-DF	Antiasthmatic	**Syrup (per 5 mL):** theophylline (32.5 mg), ephedrine sulfate (6.25 mg), hydroxyzine HCl (2.5 mg), alcohol (5%)	**2-5 yrs:** 2.5 - 5 mL tid - qid po. **5-12 yrs:** 5 mL tid - qid po.

TRADE NAME	THERAPEUTIC CATEGORY	DOSAGE FORMS AND COMPOSITION	COMMON PEDIATRIC DOSAGE
MAXITROL	Antibacterial-Corticosteroid	**Ophth Susp (per mL):** polymyxin B sulfate (10,000 Units), neomycin sulfate (equal to 3.5 mg of neomycin base), dexamethasone (0.1%)	1 or 2 drops into the affected eye(s) q 1 h in severe disease; in mild cases, 1 - 2 drops 4 to 6 times daily.
		Ophth Oint (per g): polymyxin B sulfate (10,000 Units), neomycin sulfate (equal to 3.5 mg of neomycin base), dexamethasone (0.1%)	Apply a small amount into the conjunctival sac tid to qid.
METIMYD	Antibacterial-Corticosteroid	**Ophth Susp:** sulfacetamide sodium (10%), prednisolone acetate (0.5%)	2 - 3 drops into the affected eye(s) q 1 - 2 h during the day and hs.
		Ophth Oint: sulfacetamide sodium (10%), prednisolone acetate (0.5%)	Apply to affected eye(s) tid or qid and hs.
MOBIGESIC	Non-Opioid Analgesic	**Tab:** magnesium salicylate (325 mg), phenyltoloxamine citrate (30 mg)	6-12 yrs: 1 tablet q 4 h po, up to 5 tablets daily.
MYCITRACIN PLUS PAIN RELIEVER	Antibacterial-Local Anesthetic	**Oint (per g):** polymyxin B sulfate (5,000 Units), neomycin sulfate (equal to 3.5 mg of neomycin), bacitracin (500 Units), lidocaine (40 mg)	Apply a small amount to the affected area 1 - 3 times daily.
MYCITRACIN TRIPLE ANTIBIOTIC	Antibacterial	**Oint (per g):** polymyxin B sulfate (5,000 Units), neomycin sulfate (equal to 3.5 mg of neomycin), bacitracin (500 Units)	Apply a small amount to the affected area 1 - 3 times daily.
MYCOLOG-II	Corticosteroid-Antifungal	**Cream & Oint (per g):** triamcinolone acetonide (1.0 mg), nystatin (100,000 Units)	Apply to the affected areas bid in the morning and evening.
NALDECON	Decongestant-Antihistamine	**Syrup (per 5 mL):** phenylpropanolamine HCl (20 mg), phenylephrine HCl (5 mg), phenyltoloxamine citrate (7.5 mg), chlorpheniramine maleate (2.5 mg)	6-12 yrs (over 50 lbs): 2.5 mL q 3 - 4 h po.
		Sustained-Action Tab: phenylpropanolamine HCl (40 mg), phenylephrine HCl (10 mg), phenyltoloxamine citrate (15 mg), chlorpheniramine maleate (5 mg)	6-12 yrs (over 50 lbs): 1/2 tablet on arising, in mid-afternoon, and at bedtime po.

NALDECON PEDIATRIC	Decongestant-Antihistamine	**Solution (Drops) (per mL):** phenylpropanolamine HCl (5 mg), phenylephrine HCl (1.25 mg), phenyltoloxamine citrate (2 mg), chlorpheniramine maleate (0.5 mg)	**3-6 mos (12-17 lbs):** 0.25 mL q 3 - 4 h po. **6-12 mos (17-24 lbs):** 0.5 mL q 3 - 4 h po. **1-6 yrs (24-50 lbs):** 1 mL q 3 to 4 h po.
		Syrup (per 5 mL): phenylpropanolamine HCl (5 mg), phenylephrine HCl (1.25 mg), phenyltoloxamine citrate (2 mg), chlorpheniramine maleate (0.5 mg)	**6-12 mos (17-24 lbs):** 2.5 mL q 3 - 4 h po. **1-6 yrs (24-50 lbs):** 5 mL q 3 to 4 h po. **6-12 yrs (over 50 lbs):** 10 mL q 3 - 4 h po.
NALDECON-DX CHILDREN'S	Decongestant-Expectorant-Antitussive	**Syrup (per 5 mL):** phenylpropanolamine HCl (6.25 mg), guaifenesin (100 mg), dextromethorphan HBr (5 mg), alcohol (5%)	**2-6 yrs:** 5 mL q 4 h po. **6-12 yrs:** 10 mL q 4 h po.
NALDECON-DX PEDIATRIC	Decongestant-Expectorant-Antitussive	**Solution (Drops) (per mL):** phenylpropanolamine HCl (6.25 mg), guaifenesin (50 mg), dextromethorphan HBr (5 mg), alcohol (0.6%)	**1-3 mos (8-12 lbs):** 1/4 mL q 4 h po. **4-6 mos (13-17 lbs):** 1/2 mL q 4 h po. **7-9 mos (18-20 lbs):** 3/4 mL q 4 h po. **10-24 mos (21+ lbs):** 1.0 mL q 4 h po. **2-6 yrs:** 1.0 mL q 4 h po.
NALDECON-EX CHILDREN'S	Decongestant-Expectorant	**Syrup (per 5 mL):** phenylpropanolamine HCl (6.25 mg), guaifenesin (100 mg), alcohol (5%)	**2-6 yrs:** 5 mL q 4 h po. **6-12 yrs:** 10 mL q 4 h po.
NALDECON-EX PEDIATRIC	Decongestant-Expectorant	**Solution (Drops) (per mL):** phenylpropanolamine HCl (6.25 mg), guaifenesin (50 mg), alcohol (0.6%)	**1-3 mos (8-12 lbs):** 1/4 mL q 4 h po. **4-6 mos (13-17 lbs):** 1/2 mL q 4 h po. **7-9 mos (18-20 lbs):** 3/4 mL q 4 h po. **10-24 mos (21+ lbs):** 1.0 mL q 4 h po. **2-6 yrs:** 1.0 mL q 4 h po.

TRADE NAME	THERAPEUTIC CATEGORY	DOSAGE FORMS AND COMPOSITION	COMMON PEDIATRIC DOSAGE
NAPHCON-A	Ocular Decongestant-Antihistamine	**Ophth Solution:** naphazoline HCl (0.025%), pheniramine maleate (0.3%)	Instill 1 - 2 drops in the affected eye(s) up to qid.
NASAL	Nasal Moisturizer	**Nasal Solution & Spray:** sodium chloride (0.65%), buffered with monobasic and dibasic sodium phosphate	Over 6 yrs: 2 - 6 drops or spray twice in each nostril prn.
NATURE'S REMEDY	Stimulant Laxative	**Tab:** cascara sagrada (150 mg), aloe (100 mg)	8-15 yrs: 1 tab po with a full glass of water.
NEO-DECADRON	Antibacterial-Corticosteroid	**Topical Cream:** neomycin sulfate (equal to 0.35% of base), dexamethasone sodium phosphate (0.1%)	Apply topically to the affected area as a thin film tid - qid.
NEOSPORIN	Antibacterial	**Oint (per g):** polymyxin B sulfate (5,000 Units), neomycin sulfate (equal to 3.5 mg of neomycin base), bacitracin zinc (400 Units)	Apply topically 1 - 3 times daily.
NEOSPORIN PLUS MAXIMUM STRENGTH	Antibacterial-Local Anesthetic	**Cream (per g):** polymyxin B sulfate (10,000 Units), neomycin sulfate (equal to 3.5 mg of neomycin base), pramoxine HCl (10 mg)	**Over 2 yrs:** Apply topically 1 - 3 times daily.
		Oint (per g): polymyxin B sulfate (10,000 Units), neomycin sulfate (equal to 3.5 mg of neomycin base), bacitracin zinc (500 Units), pramoxine HCl (10 mg)	**Over 2 yrs:** Apply topically 1 - 3 times daily.
NUCOFED (C-III)	Decongestant-Antitussive	**Syrup (per 5 mL):** pseudoephedrine HCl (60 mg), codeine phosphate (20 mg)	**2-6 yrs:** 1.25 mL q 6 h po. **6-12 yrs:** 2.5 mL q 6 h po.
NUCOFED EXPECTORANT (C-III)	Decongestant-Expectorant-Antitussive	**Syrup (per 5 mL):** pseudoephedrine HCl (60 mg), guaifenesin (200 mg), codeine phosphate (20 mg), alcohol (12.5%)	**2-6 yrs:** 1.25 mL q 6 h po. **6-12 yrs:** 2.5 mL q 6 h po.
NUCOFED PEDIATRIC EXPECTORANT (C-III)	Decongestant-Expectorant-Antitussive	**Syrup (per 5 mL):** pseudoephedrine HCl (30 mg), guaifenesin (100 mg), codeine phosphate (10 mg), alcohol (6%)	**2-6 yrs:** 2.5 mL q 6 h po. **6-12 yrs:** 5 mL q 6 h po.
OCUHIST	Topical Antihistamine-Ocular Decongestant	**Ophth Solution:** pheniramine maleate (0.3%), naphazoline HCl (0.025%)	Over 6 yrs: 1 - 2 drops into affected eye(s) up to qid.
ORNEX	Decongestant-Analgesic	**Cplt:** pseudoephedrine HCl (30 mg), acetaminophen (325 mg)	6-12 yrs: 1 caplet q 4 h po, not to exceed 4 caplets in 24 h.

OTOBIOTIC	Antibacterial-Corticosteroid	**Otic Solution (per mL):** polymyxin B sulfate (10,000 Units), hydrocortisone (0.5%)	3 drops into ear(s) tid or qid.
PEDIACARE COLD-ALLERGY	Decongestant-Antihistamine	**Chewable Tab:** pseudoephedrine HCl (15 mg), chlorpheniramine maleate (1 mg)	**2-3 yrs (24-35 lbs):** 1 tablet q 4 - 6 h po. **4-5 yrs (36-47 lbs):** 1.5 tablets q 4 - 6 h po. **6-8 yrs (48-59 lbs):** 2 tablets q 4 - 6 h po. **9-10 yrs (60-71 lbs):** 2.5 tablets q 4 - 6 h po. **11-12 yrs (72-95 lbs):** 3 tablets q 4 - 6 h po.
PEDIACARE COUGH-COLD	Decongestant-Antihistamine-Antitussive	**Liquid (per 5 mL):** pseudoephedrine HCl (15 mg), chlorpheniramine maleate (1 mg), dextromethorphan HBr (5 mg)	**2-3 yrs (24-35 lbs):** 5 mL q 4 to 6 h po. **4-5 yrs (36-47 lbs):** 7.5 mL q 4 - 6 h po. **6-8 yrs (48-59 lbs):** 10 mL q 4 to 6 h po. **9-10 yrs (60-71 lbs):** 12.5 mL q 4 - 6 h po. **11-12 yrs (72-95 lbs):** 15 mL q 4 - 6 h po.
		Chewable Tab: pseudoephedrine HCl (15 mg), chlorpheniramine maleate (1 mg), dextromethorphan HBr (5 mg)	**2-3 yrs (24-35 lbs):** 1 tab q 4 to 6 h po. **4-5 yrs (36-47 lbs):** 1.5 tabs q 4 to 6 h po. **6-8 yrs (48-59 lbs):** 2 tabs q 4 to 6 h po. **9-10 yrs (60-71 lbs):** 2.5 tabs q 4 - 6 h po. **11-12 yrs (72-95 lbs):** 3 tabs q 4 - 6 h po.

133

TRADE NAME	THERAPEUTIC CATEGORY	DOSAGE FORMS AND COMPOSITION	COMMON PEDIATRIC DOSAGE
PEDIACARE INFANTS' DROPS DECONGESTANT PLUS COUGH	Decongestant-Antitussive	Liquid (Drops) (per 0.8 mL): pseudoephedrine HCl (7.5 mg), dextromethorphan HBr (2.5 mg)	Birth - 3 mos (6-11 lbs): 0.4 mL q 4 - 6 h po. 4-11 mos (12-17 lbs): 0.8 mL q 4 - 6 h po. 1-2 yrs (18-23 lbs): 1.2 mL q 4 to 6 h po. 2-3 yrs (24-35 lbs): 1.6 mL q 4 to 6 h po.
PEDIACARE NIGHT-REST COUGH-COLD	Decongestant-Antihistamine-Antitussive	Liquid (per 5 mL): pseudoephedrine HCl (15 mg), chlorpheniramine maleate (1 mg), dextromethorphan HBr (7.5 mg)	2-3 yrs (24-35 lbs): 5 mL q 6 to 8 h po. 4-5 yrs (36-47 lbs): 7.5 mL q 6 to 8 h po. 6-8 yrs (48-59 lbs): 10 mL q 6 to 8 h po. 9-10 yrs (60-71 lbs): 12.5 mL q 6 - 8 h po. 11-12 yrs (72-95 lbs): 15 mL q 6 - 8 h po.
PEDIACOF (C-VI)	Decongestant-Antihistamine-Antitussive-Expectorant	Syrup (per 5 mL): phenylephrine HCl (2.5 mg), chlorpheniramine maleate (0.75 mg), codeine phosphate (5 mg), potassium iodide (75 mg), alcohol (5%)	6-12 mos: 1.25 mL q 4 - 6 h po 1-3 yrs: 2.5 - 5 mL q 4 - 6 h po. 3-6 yrs: 5 - 10 mL q 4 - 6 h po. 6-12 yrs: 10 mL q 4 - 6 h po.
PEDIAMIST	Nasal Moisturizer	Nasal Spray: sodium chloride (0.5%), water, glycerin	Infants: 1 - 2 sprays in each nostril prn. Children: Up to 4 sprays in each nostril prn.

PEDIAZOLE	Antibacterial	**Powder for Susp (per 5 mL):** erythromycin ethylsuccinate (200 mg), sulfisoxazole (600 mg).	**Over 2 mos:** 50 mg/kg/day po (based on the erythromycin content) in equally divided doses tid - qid for 10 days. **Approximate qid dosage by weight:** **8 kg (18 lbs):** 2.5 mL q 6 h po. **16 kg (35 lbs):** 5 mL q 6 h po. **24 kg (53 lbs):** 7.5 mL q 6 h po. **Over 32 kg (70 lbs):** 10 mL q 6 h po. **Approximate tid dosage by weight:** **6 kg (13 lbs):** 2.5 mL q 8 h po. **12 kg (26 lbs):** 5 mL q 8 h po. **18 kg (40 lbs):** 7.5 mL q 8 h po. **24 kg (53 lbs):** 10 mL q 8 h po. **Over 30 kg (66 lbs):** 12.5 mL q 8 h po.
PEDIOTIC	Antibacterial-Corticosteroid	**Otic Susp (per mL):** polymyxin B sulfate (10,000 Units), neomycin sulfate (equal to 3.5 mg of neomycin base), hydrocortisone (10 mg = 1%).	3 drops into the affected ear(s) tid - qid.
PERCODAN-DEMI (C-II)	Analgesic	**Tab:** oxycodone HCl (2.25 mg), oxycodone terephthalate (0.19 mg), aspirin (325 mg).	**6-12:** 1/4 tab q 6 h po, prn pain. **12 yrs and older:** 1/2 tab q 6 h po, prn pain.
PERCOGESIC	Non-Opioid Analgesic	**Tab:** acetaminophen (325 mg), phenyltoloxamine citrate (30 mg).	**6-12 yrs:** 1 tablet q 4 h po, not to exceed 4 doses daily.
PERDIEM	Bulk Laxative-Stimulant Laxative	**Granules (per rounded teaspoonful):** psyllium (3.25 g), senna (0.74 g).	**7-11 yrs:** 1 rounded teaspoonful in at least 8 oz. of cool beverage 1 - 2 times daily po.

135

TRADE NAME	THERAPEUTIC CATEGORY	DOSAGE FORMS AND COMPOSITION	COMMON PEDIATRIC DOSAGE
PERI-COLACE	Stimulant Laxative-Stool Softener	**Syrup (per 15 mL)**: casanthranol (30 mg), docusate sodium (60 mg), alcohol (10%)	5 - 15 mL daily hs po.
PHENERGAN VC	Antihistamine-Decongestant	**Syrup (per 5 mL)**: promethazine HCl (6.25 mg), phenylephrine HCl (5 mg), alcohol (7%)	**2-6 yrs:** 1.25 - 2.5 mL q 4 - 6 h po. **6-12 yrs:** 2.5 - 5 mL q 4 - 6 h po.
PHENERGAN VC W/CODEINE (C-V)	Antihistamine-Decongestant-Antitussive	**Syrup (per 5 mL)**: promethazine HCl (6.25 mg), phenylephrine HCl (5 mg), codeine phosphate (10 mg), alcohol (7%)	**2-6 yrs:** 1.25 - 2.5 mL q 4 - 6 h po. Daily maximum based on the child's weight: **12 kg or 25 lbs:** 6.0 mL. **14 kg or 30 lbs:** 7.0 mL. **16 kg or 35 lbs:** 8.0 mL. **18 kg or 40 lbs:** 9.0 mL. **6-12 yrs:** 2.5 - 5 mL q 4 - 6 h po, not to exceed 30.0 mL in 24 h.
PHENERGAN W/CODEINE (C-V)	Antihistamine-Antitussive	**Syrup (per 5 mL)**: promethazine HCl (6.25 mg), codeine phosphate (10 mg), alcohol (7%)	**2-6 yrs:** 1.25 - 2.5 mL q 4 - 6 h po. Daily maximum based on the child's weight: **12 kg or 25 lbs:** 6.0 mL. **14 kg or 30 lbs:** 7.0 mL. **16 kg or 35 lbs:** 8.0 mL. **18 kg or 40 lbs:** 9.0 mL. **6-12 yrs:** 2.5 - 5 mL q 4 - 6 h po, not to exceed 30.0 mL in 24 h.
PHENERGAN W/ DEXTROMETHORPHAN	Antihistamine-Antitussive	**Syrup (per 5 mL)**: promethazine HCl (6.25 mg), dextromethorphan HBr (15 mg), alcohol (7%)	**2-6 yrs:** 1.25 - 2.5 mL q 4 - 6 h po, not to exceed 10 mL in 24 h. **6-12 yrs:** 2.5 - 5 mL q 4 - 6 h po, not to exceed 20 mL in 24 h.

POLY-HISTINE	Antihistamine	**Elixir (per 5 mL):** pheniramine maleate (4 mg), pyrilamine maleate (4 mg), phenyltoloxamine citrate (4 mg), alcohol (4%)	**2-6 yrs:** 2.5 mL q 4 h po. **6-12 yrs:** 5 mL q 4 h po.
POLY-HISTINE-D PED CAPS	Decongestant-Antihistamine	**Timed-Rel. Cpsl:** phenylpropanolamine HCl (25 mg), pheniramine maleate (8 mg), pyrilamine maleate (8 mg), phenyltoloxamine citrate (8 mg)	**6-12 yrs:** 1 cpsl q 8 - 12 h po.
POLY-PRED	Antibacterial-Corticosteroid	**Ophth Susp (per mL):** neomycin sulfate (equal to 3.5 mg of neomycin base), polymyxin B sulfate (10,000 Units), prednisolone acetate (0.5%)	1 or 2 drops q 3 - 4 h into affected eye(s). Acute infections may require dosing q 30 minutes, initially.
POLYSPORIN	Antibacterial	**Powder & Oint (per g):** polymyxin B sulfate (10,000 Units), bacitracin zinc (500 units)	Apply topically 1 - 3 times daily.
POLYTRIM	Antibacterial	**Ophth Solution (per mL):** trimethoprim sulfate (equal to 1 mg of trimethoprim base), polymyxin B sulfate (10,000 Units)	**Over 2 mos:** 1 drop into the affected eye(s) q 3 h (maximum of 6 doses per day) for 7 - 10 days.
PRAMOSONE 1%	Corticosteroid-Local Anesthetic	**Cream, Lotion & Oint:** hydrocortisone acetate (1%), pramoxine HCl (1%)	Apply as a thin film to affected area tid - qid.
PRAMOSONE 2.5%	Corticosteroid-Local Anesthetic	**Cream, Lotion & Oint:** hydrocortisone acetate (2.5%), pramoxine HCl (1%)	Apply as a thin film to affected area tid - qid.
PREFRIN LIQUIFILM	Ocular Lubricant-Vasoconstrictor	**Ophth Sol:** polyvinyl alcohol (1.4%), phenylephrine HCl (0.12%)	1 - 2 drops into affected eye(s) up to qid.
PROCTOCREAM-HC	Local Anesthetic-Corticosteroid	**Cream:** pramoxine HCl (1%), hydrocortisone acetate (1%)	Apply to the affected area as a thin film tid - qid.
PROCTOFOAM-HC	Local Anesthetic-Corticosteroid	**Aerosol:** pramoxine HCl (1%), hydrocortisone acetate (1%)	Apply to the affected area tid to qid.

TRADE NAME	THERAPEUTIC CATEGORY	DOSAGE FORMS AND COMPOSITION	COMMON PEDIATRIC DOSAGE
PRONTO	Pediculicide	**Shampoo:** pyrethrum extract (0.33%), piperonyl butoxide (4%)	Apply to dry hair and scalp or other affected areas. Use enough to completely wet area being treated; massage in. Allow the product to remain for 10 minutes, but no longer. Rinse and towel dry. Repeat in 7 - 10 days if reinfestation occurs.
QUADRINAL	Antiasthmatic	**Tab:** theophylline calcium salicylate (130 mg; equal to 65 mg of theophylline base), ephedrine HCl (24 mg), potassium iodide (320 mg), phenobarbital (24 mg)	**6-12 yrs:** 1/2 tab tid po.
QUELIDRINE	Decongestant-Expectorant-Antitussive-Antihistamine	**Syrup (per 5 mL):** ephedrine HCl (5 mg), phenylephrine HCl (5 mg), ammonium chloride (40 mg), ipecac fluidextract (0.005 mL), dextromethorphan HBr (10 mg), chlorpheniramine maleate (2 mg), alcohol (2%)	**2-6 yrs:** 1.25 mL 1 to 4 times daily po. **6-12 yrs:** 2.5 mL 1 to 4 times daily po.
QUIBRON QUIBRON-300	Antiasthmatic	**Cpsl:** theophylline (150 mg), guaifenesin (90 mg) **Cpsl:** theophylline (300 mg), guaifenesin (180 mg)	Dose based on theophylline; see Oral Theophylline Doses Table, Section I., p. 158.
R & C	Pediculicide	**Shampoo:** pyrethrins (0.30%), piperonyl butoxide technical (3%)	Apply to dry hair and scalp or other affected areas. Use enough to completely wet area being treated; massage in. Allow the product to remain for 10 min. Rinse and towel dry. Repeat in 7 - 10 days if reinfestation occurs.
RHULIGEL	Analgesic (Topical)	**Gel:** benzyl alcohol (2.0%), camphor (0.3%), menthol (0.3%)	**Over 2 yrs:** Apply to affected areas no more than qid.
RHULISPRAY	Local Anesthetic-Skin Protectant	**Aerosol:** benzocaine (5.0%), calamine (13.8%), camphor (0.7%)	**Over 2 yrs:** Apply to affected areas no more than qid.

138

RID	Pediculicide	Shampoo: pyrethrum extract (0.33%), piperonyl butoxide technical (4%)	Apply to dry hair and scalp or other affected areas. Use enough to completely wet area being treated; massage in. Allow the product to remain for 10 min. Rinse and towel dry. Repeat in 7 - 10 days if reinfestation occurs.
ROBITUSSIN A-C (C-V)	Antitussive-Expectorant	Syrup (per 5 mL): codeine phosphate (10 mg), guaifenesin (100 mg), alcohol (3.5%)	6-12 yrs: 5 mL q 4 h po. Do not exceed 4 doses in 24 h.
ROBITUSSIN-CF	Decongestant-Expectorant-Antitussive	Liquid (per 5 mL): phenylpropanolamine HCl (12.5 mg), guaifenesin (100 mg), dextromethorphan HBr (10 mg)	2-6 yrs: 2.5 mL q 4 h po. Do not exceed 4 doses in 24 h. 6-12 yrs: 5 mL q 4 h po. Do not exceed 4 doses in 24 h.
ROBITUSSIN COLD & COUGH LIQUI-GELS	Decongestant-Expectorant-Antitussive	Softgel: pseudoephedrine HCl (30 mg), guaifenesin (200 mg), dextromethorphan HBr (10 mg)	6-12 yrs: 1 Softgel q 4 h po. Do not exceed 4 doses in 24 h.
ROBITUSSIN COLD, COUGH & FLU LIQUI-GELS	Antitussive-Decongestant-Expectorant-Analgesic	Softgel: dextromethorphan HBr (10 mg), pseudoephedrine HCl (30 mg), guaifenesin (100 mg), acetaminophen (250 mg)	6-12 yrs: 1 Softgel q 4 h po. Do not exceed 4 doses in 24 h.
ROBITUSSIN-DAC (C-V)	Decongestant-Expectorant-Antitussive	Syrup (per 5 mL): pseudoephedrine HCl (30 mg), guaifenesin (100 mg), codeine phosphate (10 mg), alcohol (1.9%)	6-12 yrs: 5 mL q 4 h po. Do not exceed 4 doses in 24 h.
ROBITUSSIN-DM	Antitussive-Expectorant	Liquid (per 5 mL): dextromethorphan HBr (10 mg), guaifenesin (100 mg)	2-6 yrs: 2.5 mL q 4 h po. Do not exceed 4 doses in 24 h. 6-12 yrs: 5 mL q 4 h po. Do not exceed 4 doses in 24 h.
ROBITUSSIN-PE	Decongestant-Expectorant	Liquid (per 5 mL): pseudoephedrine HCl (30 mg), guaifenesin (100 mg)	2-6 yrs: 2.5 mL q 4 h po. Do not exceed 4 doses in 24 h. 6-12 yrs: 5 mL q 4 h po. Do not exceed 4 doses in 24 h.

TRADE NAME	THERAPEUTIC CATEGORY	DOSAGE FORMS AND COMPOSITION	COMMON PEDIATRIC DOSAGE
ROBITUSSIN PEDIATRIC COUGH & COLD FORMULA	Decongestant-Antitussive	**Liquid (per 5 mL):** pseudoephedrine HCl (15 mg), dextromethorphan HBr (7.5 mg)	**2-6 yrs (24-47 lbs):** 5 mL q 6 h po. Do not exceed 4 doses in 24 h. **6-12 yrs (48-95 lbs):** 10 mL q 6 h po. Do not exceed 4 doses in 24 h.
ROBITUSSIN PEDIATRIC DROPS	Decongestant-Antitussive-Expectorant	**Liquid (Drops) (per 2.5 mL):** pseudoephedrine HCl (15 mg), dextromethorphan HBr (5 mg), guaifenesin (100 mg)	**2-6 yrs (24-47 lbs):** 2.5 mL q 4 h po. Do not exceed 4 doses in 24 h. **6-12 yrs (48-95 lbs):** 5 mL q 4 h po. Do not exceed 4 doses in 24 h.
ROBITUSSIN SEVERE CONGESTION LIQUI-GELS	Decongestant-Expectorant	**Liqui-Gel:** pseudoephedrine HCl (30 mg), guaifenesin (200 mg)	**6-12 yrs:** 1 Softgel q 4 h po. Do not exceed 4 doses in 24 h.
RONDEC	Decongestant-Antihistamine	**Liquid (Drops) (per mL):** pseudoephedrine HCl (25 mg), carbinoxamine maleate (2 mg)	**1-3 mos:** 0.25 mL qid po. **3-6 mos:** 0.5 mL qid po. **6-9 mos:** 0.75 mL qid po. **9-18 mos:** 1 mL qid po.
		Syrup (per 5 mL): pseudoephedrine HCl (60 mg), carbinoxamine maleate (4 mg)	**18 mos - 6 yrs:** 2.5 mL qid po. **6-12 yrs:** 5 mL qid po.
		Tab: pseudoephedrine HCl (60 mg), carbinoxamine maleate (4 mg)	**6-12 yrs:** 1 tab qid po.
RONDEC-DM	Decongestant-Antihistamine-Antitussive	**Liquid (Drops) (per mL):** pseudoephedrine HCl (25 mg), carbinoxamine maleate (2 mg), dextromethorphan HBr (4 mg)	**1-3 mos:** 0.25 mL qid po. **3-6 mos:** 0.5 mL qid po. **6-9 mos:** 0.75 mL qid po. **9-18 mos:** 1 mL qid po.
		Syrup (per 5 mL): pseudoephedrine HCl (60 mg), carbinoxamine maleate (4 mg), dextromethorphan HBr (15 mg)	**18 mos - 6 yrs:** 2.5 mL qid po. **6-12 yrs:** 5 mL qid po.

RYNA	Decongestant-Antihistamine	Liquid (per 5 mL): pseudoephedrine HCl (30 mg), chlorpheniramine maleate (2 mg).	6-12 yrs: 5 mL q 6 h po.
RYNA-C (C-V)	Antitussive-Decongestant-Antihistamine	Liquid (per 5 mL): codeine phosphate (10 mg), pseudoephedrine HCl (30 mg), chlorpheniramine maleate (2 mg).	6-12 yrs: 5 mL q 6 h po.
RYNA-CX (C-V)	Antitussive-Decongestant-Expectorant	Liquid (per 5 mL): codeine phosphate (10 mg), pseudoephedrine HCl (30 mg), guaifenesin (100 mg).	6-12 yrs: 5 mL q 6 h po.
RYNATAN PEDIATRIC	Decongestant-Antihistamine	Susp (per 5 mL): phenylephrine tannate (5 mg), pyrilamine tannate (12.5 mg), chlorpheniramine tannate (2 mg).	2-6 yrs: 2.5 - 5 mL q 12 h po. 6-12 yrs: 5 - 10 mL q 12 h po.
RYNATUSS PEDIATRIC	Decongestant-Antihistamine-Antitussive	Susp (per 5 mL): phenylephrine tannate (5 mg), chlorpheniramine tannate (4 mg), ephedrine tannate (5 mg), carbetapentane tannate (30 mg).	2-6 yrs: 2.5 - 5 mL q 12 h po. 6-12 yrs: 5 - 10 mL q 12 h po.
SENOKOT-S	Stimulant Laxative-Stool Softener	Tab: senna concentrate (8.6 mg sennosides), docusate sodium (50 mg)	2-6 yrs: 1/2 tab once daily po. 6-12 yrs: 1 tab once daily po.
SEPTRA	Antibacterial	Tab: trimethoprim (80 mg), sulfamethoxazole (400 mg) Susp & Pediatric Susp (per 5 mL): trimethoprim (40 mg), sulfamethoxazole (200 mg)	Urinary Tract Infections or Acute Otitis Media (Over 2 mos): 8 mg/kg trimethoprim and 40 mg/kg sulfamethoxazole po per 24 h, given in 2 divided doses q 12 h for 10 days. Dosage guideline (given q 12 h) based on child's weight -
SEPTRA DS		Tab: trimethoprim (160 mg), sulfamethoxazole (800 mg)	10 kg or 22 lbs: 5 mL. 20 kg or 44 lbs: 10 mL or 1 SEPTRA tablet. 30 kg or 66 lbs: 15 mL or 1.5 SEPTRA tablets. 40 kg or 88 lbs: 20 mL, 2 SEPTRA tablets, or 1 SEPTRA DS tablet.

[Continued on the next page]

TRADE NAME	THERAPEUTIC CATEGORY	DOSAGE FORMS AND COMPOSITION	COMMON PEDIATRIC DOSAGE

SEPTRA and SEPTRA DS
[Continued]

Shigellosis (Over 2 mos): Same daily dose is used for 5 days po.

Pneumocystis carinii **Pneumonia Treatment (Over 2 mos):**
15 - 20 mg/kg trimethoprim and 75 - 100 mg/kg sulfamethoxazole po per 24 h in equally divided doses q 6 h for 14 - 21 days.
Dosage guideline (given q 6 h) based on child's weight -

8 kg or 18 lbs: 5 mL.
16 kg or 35 lbs: 10 mL or 1 SEPTRA tablet.
24 kg or 53 lbs: 15 mL or 1.5 SEPTRA tablets.
32 kg or 70 lbs: 20 mL, 2 SEPTRA tablets, or 1 SEPTRA DS tablet.

Pneumocystis carinii **Pneumonia Prophylaxis (Over 2 mos):**
150 mg/m^2 trimethoprim and 750 mg/m^2 sulfamethoxazole po per 24 h in equally divided doses bid on 3 consecutive days per week. The total daily dose should not exceed 320 mg trimethoprim and 1600 mg sulfamethoxazole.
Dosage guideline based on child's body surface area -

0.26 m^2: 2.5 mL.
0.53 m^2: 5 mL or 1/2 SEPTRA tablet.
1.06 m^2: 10 mL or 1 SEPTRA tablet.

142

SEPTRA I.V. INFUSION	Antibacterial	**Inj (per 5 mL):** trimethoprim (80 mg), sulfamethoxazole (400 mg)
		Severe Urinary Tract Infections and Shigellosis (Over 2 mos): 8 - 10 mg/kg daily (based on trimethoprim) in 2 - 4 equally divided doses q 6, 8 or 12 h by IV infusion for up to 14 days for UTI and 5 days for shigellosis. ***Pneumocystis carinii* Pneumonia (Over 2 mos):** 15 - 20 mg/kg daily (based on trimethoprim) in 3 - 4 equally divided doses q 6 - 8 h by IV infusion for up to 14 days.
SINAREST	Decongestant-Analgesic-Antihistamine	**Tab:** pseudoephedrine HCl (30 mg), acetaminophen (325 mg), chlorpheniramine maleate (2 mg)
		6-12 yrs: 1 tab q 4 - 6 h po, not to exceed 4 tablets in 24 h.
SINAREST NO DROWSINESS	Decongestant-Analgesic	**Tab:** pseudoephedrine HCl (30 mg), acetaminophen (500 mg)
		6-12 yrs: 1 tab q 4 - 6 h po, not to exceed 4 tablets in 24 h.
SINULIN	Decongestant-Antihistamine-Analgesic	**Tab:** phenylpropanolamine HCl (25 mg), chlorpheniramine maleate (4 mg), acetaminophen (650 mg)
		6-12 yrs: 1/2 tab q 4 - 6 h po.
SLO-PHYLLIN GG	Antiasthmatic	**Syrup (per 15 mL):** theophylline anhydrous (150 mg), guaifenesin (90 mg) **Cpsl:** theophylline anhydrous (150 mg), guaifenesin (90 mg)
		Dose based on theophylline; see the Theophylline Table, Section I, p. 158.
ST. JOSEPH COLD TABLETS	Decongestant-Analgesic	**Chewable Tab:** phenylpropanolamine HCl (3.125 mg), acetaminophen (80 mg)
		2-3 yrs (27-35 lbs): 2 tabs q 4 h po. **4-5 yrs (36-45 lbs):** 3 tabs q 4 h po. **6-8 yrs (46-65 lbs):** 4 tabs q 4 h po. **9-10 yrs (66-76 lbs):** 5 tabs q 4 h po. **11-12 yrs (77-83 lbs):** 6 tabs q 4 h po. **12+ yrs (83+ lbs):** 8 tabs q 4 h po.

143

TRADE NAME	THERAPEUTIC CATEGORY	DOSAGE FORMS AND COMPOSITION	COMMON PEDIATRIC DOSAGE
SUDAFED COLD & ALLERGY	Decongestant-Antihistamine	**Tab:** pseudoephedrine HCl (60 mg), chlorpheniramine maleate (4 mg)	**6-12 yrs:** 1/2 tab q 4 - 6 h po, not to exceed 4 doses in 24 h.
SUDAFED COUGH & COLD, CHILDREN'S	Decongestant-Antitussive	**Liquid (per 5 mL):** pseudoephedrine HCl (15 mg), dextromethorphan HBr (5 mg)	**2-6 yrs:** 5 mL q 4 h po, not to exceed 4 doses in 24 h. **6-12 yrs:** 10 mL q 4 h po, not to exceed 4 doses in 24 h.
TERRA-CORTRIL	Antibacterial-Corticosteroid	**Ophth Susp (per mL):** oxytetracycline (5 mg), hydrocortisone acetate (15 mg)	1 or 2 drops into the affected eye(s) tid.
TERRAMYCIN	Antibacterial	**Inj (per mL):** oxytetracycline (50 mg), lidocaine (2%) **Inj (per mL):** oxytetracycline (125 mg), lidocaine (2%)	**Over 8 yrs:** 15 - 25 mg/kg/day IM in divided doses q 8 - 12 h.
		Ophth Oint (per g): oxytetracycline (5 mg), polymyxin B sulfate (10,000 units)	Apply approx. 1/2 in onto the lower lid of the affected eye(s) bid - qid.
THYROLAR 1/4	Thyroid Hormone	**Tab:** levothyroxine sodium (12.5 μg), liothyronine sodium (3.1 μg)	Dosage based on levothyroxine content po: **Under 6 mos:** 8 - 10 μg/kg/day. **6-12 mos:** 6 - 8 μg/kg/day. **1-5 yrs:** 5 - 6 μg/kg/day. **6-12 yrs:** 4 - 5 μg/kg/day. **Over 12 yrs:** 2 - 3 μg/kg/day.
THYROLAR 1/2		**Tab:** levothyroxine sodium (25 μg), liothyronine sodium (6.25 μg)	
THYROLAR 1		**Tab:** levothyroxine sodium (50 μg), liothyronine sodium (12.5 μg)	
THYROLAR 2		**Tab:** levothyroxine sodium (100 μg), liothyronine sodium (25 μg)	
THYROLAR 3		**Tab:** levothyroxine sodium (150 μg), liothyronine sodium (37.5 μg)	

144

Drug	Category	Formulation	Dosage

TIMENTIN	Antibacterial	**Powd for Inj:** 3.1 g (3 g ticarcillin, 0.1 g clavulanic acid)
		Powd for Inj: 3.2 g (3 g ticarcillin, 0.2 g clavulanic acid)
			Over 3 mos:
			Mild to Moderate Infections:
			  < 60 kg: 200 mg/kg/day q 6 h by IV infusion.
			  ≥ 60 kg: 3.1 g q 6 h by IV infusion.
			Severe Infections:
			  < 60 kg: 300 mg/kg/day q 4 h by IV infusion.
			  ≥ 60 kg: 3.1 g q 4 h by IV infusion.

TRIAMINIC ALLERGY	Decongestant-Antihistamine	**Tab:** phenylpropanolamine HCl (25 mg), chlorpheniramine maleate (4 mg)	**6-12 yrs:** 1/2 tablet q 4 h po.
TRIAMINIC AM COUGH AND DECONGESTANT FORMULA	Antitussive-Decongestant	**Liquid (per 5 mL):** dextromethorphan HBr (7.5 mg), pseudoephedrine HCl (15 mg)	**4-12 mos (12-17 lbs):** 1.25 mL q 6 h po. **12-24 mos (18-23 lbs):** 2.5 mL q 6 h po. **2-6 yrs (24-47 lbs):** 5 mL q 6 h po. **6-12 yrs (48-95 lbs):** 10 mL q 6 h po. **12 yrs & over (96+ lbs):** 20 mL q 6 h po.
TRIAMINIC COLD TABLETS	Decongestant-Antihistamine	**Tab:** phenylpropanolamine HCl (12.5 mg), chlorpheniramine maleate (2 mg)	**6-12 yrs:** 1 tablet q 4 h po.
TRIAMINIC-DM	Decongestant-Antitussive	**Syrup (per 5 mL):** phenylpropanolamine HCl (6.25 mg), dextromethorphan HBr (5 mg)	**4-12 mos (12-17 lbs):** 1.25 mL q 4 h po. **1-2 yrs (18-23 lbs):** 2.5 mL q 4 h po. **2-6 yrs (24-47 lbs):** 5 mL q 4 h po. **6-12 yrs (48-95 lbs):** 10 mL q 4 h po.

145

TRADE NAME	THERAPEUTIC CATEGORY	DOSAGE FORMS AND COMPOSITION	COMMON PEDIATRIC DOSAGE
TRIAMINIC EXPECTORANT	Decongestant-Expectorant	Liquid (per 5 mL): phenylpropanolamine HCl (6.25 mg), guaifenesin (50 mg), alcohol (5%)	**4-12 mos (12-17 lbs):** 1.25 mL q 4 h po. **1-2 yrs (18-23 lbs):** 2.5 mL q 4 h po. **2-6 yrs (24-47 lbs):** 5 mL q 4 h po. **6-12 yrs (48-95 lbs):** 10 mL q 4 h po.
TRIAMINIC EXPECTORANT DH (C-III)	Decongestant-Expectorant-Antitussive-Antihistamine	Liquid (per 5 mL): phenylpropanolamine HCl (12.5 mg), guaifenesin (100 mg), hydrocodone bitartrate (1.67 mg), pyrilamine maleate (6.25 mg), pheniramine maleate (6.25 mg), alcohol (5%)	**1-6 yrs:** 2.5 mL q 4 h po. **6-12 yrs:** 5 mL q 4 h po.
TRIAMINIC EXPECTORANT W/CODEINE (C-V)	Decongestant-Expectorant-Antitussive	Liquid (per 5 mL): phenylpropanolamine HCl (12.5 mg), guaifenesin (100 mg), codeine phosphate (10 mg), alcohol (5%)	**6-12 yrs:** 5 mL q 4 h po.
TRIAMINIC NIGHT TIME	Decongestant-Antihistamine-Antitussive	Liquid (per 5 mL): pseudoephedrine HCl (15 mg), chlorpheniramine maleate (1 mg), dextromethorphan HBr (7.5 mg)	**4-12 mos (12-17 lbs):** 1.25 mL q 6 h po. **1-2 yrs (18-23 lbs):** 2.5 mL q 6 h po. **2-6 yrs (24-47 lbs):** 5 mL q 6 h po. **6-12 yrs (48-95 lbs):** 10 mL q 6 h po.
TRIAMINIC ORAL INFANT	Decongestant-Antihistamine	Solution (Drops) (per mL): phenylpropanolamine HCl (20 mg), pheniramine maleate (10 mg)	1 drop/2 lbs qid po.
TRIAMINIC SORE THROAT FORMULA	Decongestant-Antitussive-Analgesic	Liquid (per 5 mL): pseudoephedrine HCl (15 mg), dextromethorphan HBr (7.5 mg), acetaminophen (160 mg)	**4-12 mos (12-17 lbs):** 1.25 mL q 6 h po. **1-2 yrs (18-23 lbs):** 2.5 mL q 6 h po. **2-6 yrs (24-47 lbs):** 5 mL q 6 h po. **6-12 yrs (48-95 lbs):** 10 mL q 6 h po.

TRIAMINIC SYRUP	Decongestant-Antihistamine	**Syrup (per 5 mL):** phenylpropanolamine HCl (6.25 mg), chlorpheniramine maleate (1 mg)	**4-12 mos (12-17 lbs):** 1.25 mL q 4 - 6 h po. **1-2 yrs (18-23 lbs):** 2.5 mL q 4 - 6 h po. **2-6 yrs (24-47 lbs):** 5 mL q 4 - 6 h po. **6-12 yrs (48-95 lbs):** 10 mL q 4 - 6 h po.
TRIAMINICOL COLD & COUGH	Decongestant-Antihistamine-Antitussive	**liquid (5 mL):** phenylpropanolamine HCl (6.25 mg), chlorpheniramine maleate (1 mg), dextromethorphan HBr (5 mg)	**4-12 mos (12-17 lbs):** 1.25 mL q 4 - 6 h po. **1-2 yrs (18-23 lbs):** 2.5 mL q 4 - 6 h po. **2-6 yrs (24-47 lbs):** 5 mL q 4 - 6 h po. **6-12 yrs (48-95 lbs):** 10 mL q 4 - 6 h po.
TRIAMINICOL MULTI-SYMPTOM COLD TABLETS	Decongestant-Antihistamine-Antitussive	**Tab:** phenylpropanolamine HCl (12.5 mg), chlorpheniramine maleate (2 mg), dextromethorphan HBr (10 mg)	**6-12 yrs:** 1 tab q 4 h po.
TRILISATE	Non-Opioid Analgesic, Antiinflammatory	**Liquid (per 5 mL):** choline magnesium salicylate (500 mg as: choline salicylate (293 mg) and magnesium salicylate (362 mg)) **Tab:** choline magnesium salicylate (500 mg as: choline salicylate (293 mg) and magnesium salicylate (362 mg)) **Tab:** choline magnesium salicylate (750 mg as: choline salicylate (440 mg) and magnesium salicylate (544 mg)) **Tab:** choline magnesium salicylate (1000 mg as: choline salicylate (587 mg) and magnesium salicylate (725 mg))	**Pain and Inflammation:** 50 mg/kg po. The total doses shown below should be given in divided doses (bid) po. **12-13 kg:** 500 mg **14-17 kg:** 750 mg **18-22 kg:** 1000 mg **23-27 kg:** 1250 mg **28-32 kg:** 1500 mg **33-37 kg:** 1750 mg **Over 37 kg:** 2250 mg
TUSSAR-DM	Decongestant-Antihistamine-Antitussive	**Liquid (per 5 mL):** pseudoephedrine HCl (30 mg), chlorpheniramine maleate (2 mg), dextromethorphan HBr (15 mg)	**6-12 yrs:** 5 mL q 6 - 8 h po.

TRADE NAME	THERAPEUTIC CATEGORY	DOSAGE FORMS AND COMPOSITION	COMMON PEDIATRIC DOSAGE
TUSSEND (C-III)	Decongestant-Antihistamine-Antitussive	**Syrup (per 5 mL):** pseudoephedrine HCl (30 mg), chlorpheniramine maleate (2 mg), hydrocodone bitartrate (2.5 mg), alcohol (5%)	**6-12 yrs:** 5 mL q 4 - 6 h po.
TUSSEND EXPECTORANT (C-III)	Decongestant-Expectorant-Antitussive	**Syrup (per 5 mL):** pseudoephedrine HCl (30 mg), guaifenesin (100 mg), hydrocodone bitartrate (2.5 mg), alcohol (5%)	**6-12 yrs:** 5 mL q 4 - 6 h po.
TUSSIONEX (C-III)	Antihistamine-Antitussive	**Extended-Rel. Susp (per 5 mL):** chlorpheniramine polistirex (8 mg), hydrocodone polistirex (10 mg)	**6-12 yrs:** 2.5 mL q 12 h po.
TUSSI-ORGANIDIN NR (C-V)	Antitussive-Expectorant	**Liquid (per 5 mL):** codeine phosphate (10 mg), guaifenesin (100 mg)	**2-6 yrs:** 1 mg/kg/day of codeine po in 4 equally divided doses. **6-12 yrs:** 5 mL q 4 h po.
TUSSI-ORGANIDIN DM NR	Antitussive-Expectorant	**Liquid (per 5 mL):** dextromethorphan HBr (10 mg), guaifenesin (100 mg)	**2-6 yrs:** 2.5 mL q 4 h po. **6-12 yrs:** 5 mL q 4 h po.
TYLENOL ALLERGY-D, CHILDREN'S	Analgesic-Antihistamine-Decongestant	**Liquid (per 5 mL):** acetaminophen (160 mg), diphenhydramine HCl (12.5 mg), pseudoephedrine HCl (15 mg) **Chewable Tablets:** acetaminophen (80 mg), diphenhydramine HCl (6.25 mg), pseudoephedrine HCl (7.5 mg)	**6-11 yrs (48-95 lbs):** 10 mL q 4 - 6 h po. **6-11 yrs (48-95 lbs):** Chew 4 tabs q 4 - 6 h po.
TYLENOL COLD, CHILDREN'S	Analgesic/Antipyretic-Antihistamine-Decongestant	**Liquid (per 5 mL):** acetaminophen (160 mg), chlorpheniramine maleate (1 mg), pseudoephedrine HCl (15 mg) **Chewable Tab:** acetaminophen (80 mg), chlorpheniramine maleate (0.5 mg), pseudoephedrine HCl (7.5 mg)	**2-5 yrs (24-47 lbs):** 5 mL q 4 - 6 h po. **6-11 yrs (48-95 lbs):** 10 mL q 4 - 6 h po. Do not exceed 4 doses in 24 h. **2-5 yrs (24-47 lbs):** 2 tabs q 4 - 6 h po. **6-11 yrs (48-95 lbs):** 4 tabs q 4 - 6 h po. Do not exceed 4 doses in 24 h.

TYLENOL COLD, INFANT'S	Antipyretic-Decongestant	**Liquid (Drops) (per 0.8 mL):** acetaminophen (80 mg), pseudoephedrine HCl (7.5 mg)	**Birth - 3 mos (6-11 lbs):** 0.4 mL q 4 - 6 h po. **4-11 mos (12-17 lbs):** 0.8 mL q 4 - 6 h po. **12-23 mos (18-23 lbs):** 1.2 mL q 4 - 6 h po. **2-3 yrs (24-35 lbs):** 1.6 mL q 4 - 6 h po. Do not exceed 4 doses in 24 h. **6-11 yrs:** 1 cplt (or tab) q 6 h po.
TYLENOL COLD MEDICATION, MULTI-SYMPTOM	Analgesic-Antihistamine-Decongestant-Antitussive	**Cplt & Tab:** acetaminophen (325 mg), chlorpheniramine maleate (2 mg), pseudoephedrine HCl (30 mg), dextromethorphan HBr (15 mg)	**6-11 yrs:** 1 cplt (or gelcap) q 6 h po.
TYLENOL COLD MEDICATION, NO DROWSINESS FORMULA	Analgesic-Decongestant-Antitussive	**Cplt & Gelcap:** acetaminophen (325 mg), pseudoephedrine HCl (30 mg), dextromethorphan HBr (15 mg)	**2-5 yrs (24-47 lbs):** 5 mL q 4 - 6 h po. **6-11 yrs (48=95 lbs):** 10 mL q 4 - 6 h po. Do not exceed 4 doses in 24 h.
TYLENOL COLD PLUS COUGH, CHILDREN'S	Analgesic/Antipyretic-Antihistamine-Decongestant-Antitussive	**Liquid (per 5 mL):** acetaminophen (160 mg), chlorpheniramine maleate (1 mg), pseudoephedrine HCl (15 mg), dextromethorphan HBr (5 mg) **Chewable Tab:** acetaminophen (80 mg), chlorpheniramine maleate (0.5 mg), pseudoephedrine HCl (7.5 mg), dextromethorphan HBr (2.5 mg)	**2-5 yrs (24-47 lbs):** 5 mL q 4 - 6 h po. **6-11 yrs (48-95 lbs):** 10 mL q 4 - 6 h po. Do not exceed 4 doses in 24 h. **6-11 yrs:** 1 cplt q 6 - 8 h po.
TYLENOL COLD SEVERE CONGESTION	Analgesic-Decongestant-Antitussive-Expectorant	**Cplt:** acetaminophen (325 mg), pseudoephedrine HBr (15 mg), dextromethorphan HBr (15 mg) guaifenesin (200 mg)	
TYLENOL COUGH MEDICATION	Analgesic-Antitussive	**Liquid (per 7.5 mL):** acetaminophen (325 mg), dextromethorphan HBr (15 mg)	**6-11 yrs:** 7.5 mL q 6 - 8 h po.

TRADE NAME	THERAPEUTIC CATEGORY	DOSAGE FORMS AND COMPOSITION	COMMON PEDIATRIC DOSAGE
TYLENOL COUGH MEDICATION W/ DECONGESTANT	Analgesic-Antitussive-Decongestant	Liquid (per 7.5 mL): acetaminophen (325 mg), dextromethorphan HBr (15 mg), pseudoephedrine HCl (30 mg)	6-11 yrs: 7.5 mL q 6 - 8 h po.
TYLENOL FLU, CHILDREN'S	Analgesic/Antipyretic-Antihistamine-Decongestant-Antitussive	Liquid (per 5 mL): acetaminophen (160 mg), chlorpheniramine maleate (1 mg), pseudoephedrine HCl (15 mg), dextromethorphan HBr (7.5 mg)	2-5 yrs (24-47 lbs): 5 mL q 6 - 8 h po. 6-11 yrs (48-95 lbs): 10 mL q 6 - 8 h po.
TYLENOL SINUS, CHILDREN'S	Analgesic-Decongestant	Liquid (per 5 mL): acetaminophen (160 mg), pseudoephedrine HCl (15 mg)	2-5 yrs (24-47 lbs): 5 mL q 4 - 6 h po. 6-11 yrs (48-95 lbs): 10 mL q 4 - 6 h po.
		Chewable Tablets: acetaminophen (80 mg), pseudoephedrine HCl (7.5 mg)	2-5 yrs (24-47 lbs): Chew 2 tabs q 4 - 6 h po. 6-11 yrs (48-95 lbs): Chew 4 tabs q 4 - 6 h po. Do not exceed 4 doses in 24 h.
TYLENOL W/CODEINE (C-V)	Analgesic	Elixir (per 5 mL): acetaminophen (120 mg), codeine phosphate (12 mg), alcohol (7%)	3-6 yrs: 5 mL tid or qid po. 7-12 yrs: 10 mL tid or qid po.
TYLENOL W/CODEINE #2 (C-III) #3 (C-III) #4 (C-III)	Analgesic	Tab: acetaminophen (300 mg), codeine phosphate (15 mg) Tab: acetaminophen (300 mg), codeine phosphate (30 mg) Tab: acetaminophen (300 mg), codeine phosphate (60 mg)	Over 3 yrs: based on a codeine phosphate dose of 0.5 mg/kg po, up to q 4 h
UNASYN	Antibacterial	Powd for Inj: 1.5 g (1 g ampicillin sodium, 0.5 g subactam sodium) Powd for Inj: 3.0 g (2 g ampicillin sodium, 1 g subactam sodium)	Dose is given as the ampicillin component. Over 1 yr (< 40 kg): 300 mg/kg daily by slow IV injection (over at least 10 - 15 min) in equally divided doses q 6 h. The usual max. is 14 days. Over 1 yrs (> 40 kg): Use adult dosage.

VASOCIDIN	Antibacterial-Corticosteroid	**Ophth Solution:** sulfacetamide sodium (10%), prednisolone sodium phosphate (0.25%)	**Over 6 yrs:** 2 drops into the affected eye(s) q 4 h. Prolong dosing interval as the condition improves.
		Ophth Oint: sulfacetamide sodium (10%), prednisolone acetate (0.5%)	**Over 6 yrs:** Apply to affected eye(s) tid or qid during the day and 1 - 2 times at night.
VICKS 44D	Decongestant-Antitussive	**Liquid (per 15 mL):** pseudoephedrine HCl (60 mg), dextromethorphan HBr (30 mg), alcohol (5%)	**6-11 yrs (48-95 lbs):** 7.5 mL q 6 h po. **12 yrs and older (over 95 lbs):** 15 mL q 6 h po.
VICKS 44E	Expectorant-Antitussive	**Liquid (per 15 mL):** guaifenesin (200 mg), dextromethorphan HBr (20 mg), alcohol (5%)	**6-11 yrs (48-95 lbs):** 7.5 mL q 4 h po. **12 yrs and older (over 95 lbs):** 15 mL q 4 h po.
VICKS 44e, PEDIATRIC	Antitussive-Expectorant	**Liquid (per 15 mL):** dextromethorphan HBr (10 mg), guaifenesin (100 mg)	**6-11 mos (17-21 lbs):** 5 mL q 4 h po. **12-23 mos (22-27 lbs):** 6.25 mL q 4 h po. **2-5 yrs (28-47 lbs):** 7.5 mL q 4 h po. **6-11 yrs (48-95 lbs):** 15 mL q 4 h po. **12 yrs and older (over 95 lbs):** 30 mL q 4 h po.
VICKS 44m, PEDIATRIC	Decongestant-Antitussive-Antihistamine	**Liquid (per 15 mL):** pseudoephedrine HCl (30 mg), dextromethorphan HBr (15 mg), chlorpheniramine maleate (2 mg)	**6-11 mos (17-21 lbs):** 5 mL q 6 h po. **12-23 mos (22-27 lbs):** 6.25 mL q 6 h po. **2-5 yrs (28-47 lbs):** 7.5 mL q 6 h po. **6-11 yrs (48-95 lbs):** 15 mL q 6 h po. **12 yrs and older (over 95 lbl):** 30 mL q 6 h po.

151

TRADE NAME	THERAPEUTIC CATEGORY	DOSAGE FORMS AND COMPOSITION	COMMON PEDIATRIC DOSAGE
VICKS DAYQUIL	Decongestant-Antitussive-Analgesic	Liquid (per 30 mL): pseudoephedrine HCl (60 mg), dextromethorphan HBr (20 mg), acetaminophen (650 mg)	**6-11 yrs**: 15 mL q 4 h po, not to exceed 4 doses in 24 h. **12 yrs and older**: 30 mL q 4 h po, not to exceed 4 doses in 24 h.
		Liquicap: pseudoephedrine HCl (30 mg), dextromethorphan HBr (10 mg), acetaminophen (250 mg)	**6-11 yrs**: 1 Liquicap q 4 h po, not to exceed 4 caps in 24 h. **12 yrs and older**: 2 Liquicaps q 4 h po, not to exceed 4 doses in 24 h.
VICKS NYQUIL, CHILDREN'S	Decongestant-Antitussive-Antihistamine	Liquid (per 15 mL): pseudoephedrine HCl (30 mg), dextromethorphan HBr (15 mg), chlorpheniramine maleate (2 mg)	**6-11 yrs (48-95 lbs)**: 15 mL q 6 h po. **12 yrs and older (over 95 lbs)**: 30 mL q 6 h po.
VICODIN TUSS (C-III)	Antitussive-Expectorant	Syrup (per 5 mL): hydrocodone bitartrate (5 mg), guaifenesin (100 mg)	**6-12 yrs**: 2.5 mL po after meals and hs (not less than 4 hours apart).
VISINE A.C.	Ocular Decongestant-Ocular Astringent	Ophth Solution: tetrahydrozoline HCl (0.25%), zinc sulfate (0.25%)	**Over 6 yrs**: 1 - 2 drops into the affected eye(s) up to qid.
VISINE MOISTURIZING	Ocular Decongestant-Ocular Lubricant	Ophth Solution: tetrahydrozoline HCl (0.05%), polyethylene glycol 400 (1%)	**Over 6 yrs**: 1 - 2 drops in the affected eye(s) up to qid.
ZIRADRYL	Antihistamine-Skin Protectant	Lotion: diphenhydramine HCl (1%), zinc oxide (2%)	**Over 6 yrs**: Apply to the affected areas not more than tid or qid.

(C-II): Controlled substance, Schedule II.

(C-III): Controlled substance, Schedule III.

(C-V): Controlled substance, Schedule V.

SPECIAL

DOSAGE

TABLES

ESTIMATION OF PEDIATRIC DOSES

The most reliable source of pediatric dose information is usually the pharmaceutical company's package insert. In the absence of a specific recommended pediatric dose, an approximation can be made by several methods based on a child's age, weight or body surface area.

YOUNG'S RULE

(used to calculate dose based on AGE; for children 2 years or older):

$$Dose = Adult \ dose \times \frac{Age \ (years)}{Age + 12}$$

CLARK'S RULE

(used to calculate dose based on WEIGHT; for children 2 years or older):

$$Dose = Adult \ dose \times \frac{Weight \ (kg)}{70}$$

$$Dose = Adult \ dose \times \frac{Weight \ (lb)}{150}$$

Doses of some drugs are prescribed based on the surface area of the patient. To assist in the determination of a patient's surface area, a nomogram relating a child's height and weight is shown on the following page.

These formulas are not exact and should never be used if the pharmaceutical manufacturer provides a pediatric dose for the drug. When pediatric doses are calculated by any method, the pediatric dose should never exceed the recommended adult dose.

SURFACE AREA NOMOGRAM

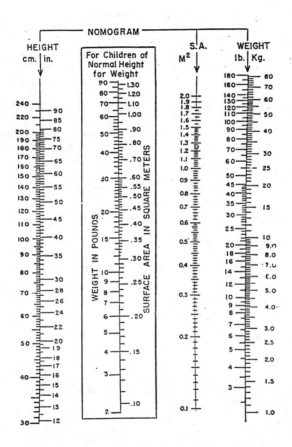

The surface area of the patient is indicated where a straight line connecting the **HEIGHT** and **WEIGHT** intersects the surface area column (**S.A.**), or if the patient is roughly of average size, from the **WEIGHT** alone (box enclosed area).

ASPIRIN DOSES BY AGE, WEIGHT AND PREPARATION

AGE (Years)	APPROXIMATE WEIGHT (Pounds)	CHEWABLE TABLETS (81 mg)[a]	ADULT TABS and CAPLETS (325 mg)[a,b]
Up to 2	Under 32	N.R.[c]	N.R.
2 to under 4	32 to 35	2	0.5
4 to under 6	36 to 45	3	0.75
6 to under 9	46 to 65	4	1
9 to under 11	66 to 76	4 - 5	1
11 to under 12	77 to 83	4 - 6	1 - 1.5
12 and Over	84 and Over	5 - 8	1 - 2

[a] Number of tablets or caplets q 4 h po.

[b] Although not recommended for use in children under 12 years, the doses listed are approximate mg equivalents of the those found in chewable tablets and these amounts have been used under supervision by a physician.

[c] Not recommended for use in this age group.

NOTE: Children and teenagers should not use aspirin for chicken pox or flu symptoms before a doctor is consulted about Reye Syndrome, a rare but serious illness.

ORAL DIGOXIN DOSES BY AGE AND PREPARATION

AGE	ELIXIR PEDIATRIC		TABLETS		CAPSULES	
	DIGITALIZING DOSE (µg/kg po)	DAILY MAINTENANCE DOSE (µg/kg po)	DIGITALIZING DOSE (µg/kg po)	DAILY MAINTENANCE DOSE (µg/kg po)	DIGITALIZING DOSE (µg/kg po)	DAILY MAINTENANCE DOSE (µg/kg po)
Premature	20 - 30	20 - 30% of the oral loading dose	Not recommended		Not recommended	
Full Term	25 - 35	25 - 35% of the oral loading dose	Not recommended	25 - 35% of the oral loading dose	Not recommended	25 - 35% of the oral or IV loading dose
1 to 24 mos	35 - 60		Not recommended		Not recommended	
2 to 5 yrs	30 - 40		30 - 40		25 - 35	
5 - 10 yrs	20 - 35		20 - 35		15 - 30	
Over 10 yrs	10 - 15		10 - 15		8 - 12	

INJECTABLE DIGOXIN DOSES BY AGE AND PREPARATION

AGE	PEDIATRIC INJECTION (100 µg/mL)		INJECTION (250 µg/mL)	
	DIGITALIZING DOSE (µg/kg IV)	DAILY MAINTENANCE DOSE (µg/kg IV)	DIGITALIZING DOSE (µg/kg IV)	DAILY MAINTENANCE DOSE (µg/kg IV)
Premature	15 - 25	20 - 30% of the IV loading dose	Not recommended	
Full Term	20 - 30	25 - 35% of the IV loading dose	Not recommended	25 - 35% of the IV loading dose
1 to 24 mos	30 - 50		Not recommended	
2 to 5 yrs	25 - 35		25 - 35	
5 - 10 yrs	15 - 30		15 - 30	
Over 10 yrs	8 - 12		8 - 12	

For all digoxin preparations, divided daily dosing is recommended for children under 10 years of age.

ORAL THEOPHYLLINE DOSES

I. **IMMEDIATE-RELEASE PREPARATIONS** (e.g., ELIXOPHYLLIN Elixir and Capsules, ELIXOPHYLLIN-GG Liquid, QUIBRON Capsules, QUIBRON-300 Capsules, SLO-PHYLLIN Syrup and Tablets, SLO-PHYLLIN GG Capsules and Syrup, and THEOLAIR Liquid and Tablets) -

Acute Symptoms of Bronchospasm Requiring Rapid Attainment of Theophylline Serum Levels for Bronchodilation -

1 - under 9 years: 5 mg/kg po (oral loading dose); then, 4 mg/kg q 6 h po (maintenance doses).
9 - under 16 years: 5 mg/kg po (oral loading dose); then, 3 mg/kg q 6 h po (maintenance doses).

Chronic Therapy -

Under 1 year: Sufficient numbers of infants under the age of 1 year have not been studied in clinical trials to support use in this age group. A physician using theophylline in this age group should carefully consider the associated benefits and risks. If used, the maintenance dose must be conservative and in accord with the following guidelines:

Premature Infants: Up to 24 days postnatal age: 1.0 mg/kg q 12 h po.
Over 24 days postnatal age: 1.5 mg/kg q 12 h po.

Infants 6 - 52 weeks: The 24 hour oral dose in mg = [(0.2 x age in weeks) + 5.0] x kg of body weight.

Up to 26 weeks: Divide the total daily dose into q 8 h dosing intervals.
26 - 52 weeks: Divide the total daily dose into q 6 h dosing intervals.

Final dosage should be guided by the serum concentration after a steady state (no further accumulation of drug) has been achieved.

Over 1 year: Initial Dose: 16 mg/kg/24 h or 400 mg/24 h (whichever is less) in divided doses q 6 - 8 h po.

Increasing Dose: The doses may be increased in approximately 25% increments at 3 day intervals, as long as the drug is tolerated, until the clinical response is satisfactory, or the maximum dose is reached.

Maximum Doses: 1 - under 9 years: 24 mg/kg/day po   12 - under 16 years: 18 mg/kg/day po
9 - under 12 years: 20 mg/kg/day po   16 years or older: 13 mg/kg/day po
not to exceed the above or 900 mg/day, whichever is less

II. SUSTAINED-RELEASE PREPARATIONS -

A. RESPBID Sustained-Release Tablets, SLO-BID Extended-Release Capsules, SLO-PHYLLIN Extended-Release Capsules, and THEOLAIR-SR Sustained-Release Tablets -

Under 6 years old or under 25 kg of body weight: Safety and efficacy have not been established. In most cases it is recommended that an immediate-release liquid preparation be used for these children.

Over 6 years old or over 25 kg of body weight:

Initial Therapy: 16 mg/kg/24 h or 400 mg/24 h (whichever is less) in 2 or 3 equally divided doses at 8 or 12 h intervals po.

Maintenance Therapy: The dose may be increased in approximately 25% increments at 3 day intervals, as long as the drug is tolerated, until the clinical response is satisfactory, or the maximum dose is reached.

Maximum Doses: 6 - under 9 years: 24 mg/kg/day po 12 - under 16 years: 18 mg/kg/day po
9 - under 12 years: 20 mg/kg/day po 16 years or older: 13 mg/kg/day po

not to exceed the above or 900 mg/day, whichever is less

B. THEO-DUR Extended-Release Tablets -

Under 6 years old or under 25 kg of body weight: Dosing of q 12 h in children under 6 has not been established. In most cases it is recommended that an immediate-release liquid preparation be used for these children.

Over 6 years old or over 25 kg of body weight:

Initial Therapy: 200 mg q 12 h po

Maintenance Therapy: The dose may be increased in approximately 25% increments at 3 day intervals, as long as the drug is tolerated, until the clinical response is satisfactory, or the maximum dose is reached.

Maximum Doses: 25 - 35 kg of body weight: 250 mg q 12 h po
35 - 70 kg of body weight: 300 mg q 12 h po

159

ORAL AMINOPHYLLINE DOSES

1.16 mg of aminophylline anhydrous = 1.0 mg of theophylline anhydrous

Acute Symptoms of Bronchospasm Requiring Rapid Attainment of Theophylline Serum Levels for Bronchodilation -

1 - under 9 years: 5.8 mg/kg po (oral loading dose); then, 4.64 mg/kg q 6 h po (maintenance doses).
9 - under 16 years: 5.8 mg/kg po (oral loading dose); then, 3.48 mg/kg q 6 h po (maintenance doses).

Chronic Therapy -

Under 1 year: Sufficient numbers of infants under the age of 1 year have not been studied in clinical trials to support use in this age group. A physician using aminophylline in this age group should carefully consider the associated benefits and risks. If used, the maintenance dose must be conservative and in accord with the following guidelines:

Premature Infants: Up to 24 days postnatal age: 1.16 mg/kg q 12 h po.
Over 24 days postnatal age: 1.74 mg/kg q 12 h po.

Infants 6 - 52 weeks: The 24 hour oral dose in mg = [(0.2 × age in weeks) + 5.8 l × kg body weight.

Up to 26 weeks: Divide the total daily dose into q 8 h dosing intervals.
26 - 52 weeks: Divide the total daily dose into q 6 h dosing intervals.

Final dosage should be guided by the serum concentration after a steady state (no further accumulation of drug) has been achieved.

Over 1 year: Initial Dose: 18.56 mg/kg/24 h or 464 mg/24 h (whichever is less) in divided doses q 6 - 8 h po.

Increasing Dose: The doses may be increased in approximately 25% increments at 3 day intervals, as long as the drug is tolerated, until the clinical response is satisfactory, or the maximum dose is reached.

Maximum Doses: 1 - under 9 years: 27.8 mg/kg/day po   12 - under 16 years: 20.88 mg/kg/day po
9 - under 12 years: 23.3 mg/kg/day po   16 years or older: 15.08 mg/kg/day po

or 1044 mg/day, whichever is less

IV AMINOPHYLLINE DOSES[a]

AGE	IV LOADING DOSE:[b]	DOSE FOR NEXT 12 HOURS:	DOSE BEYOND 12 HOURS:	MAXIMUM DAILY DOSE:
6 months to 9 years	6 mg/kg (5.16 mg/kg)	1.2 mg/kg/hr (1.03 mg/kg/hr)	1.0 mg/kg/hr (0.86 mg/kg/hr)	Variable; monitor blood levels and maintain below 20 µg/mL
9 to 16 years	6 mg/kg (5.16 mg/kg)	1.0 mg/kg/hr (0.86 mg/kg/hr)	0.8 mg/kg/hr (0.69 mg/kg/hr)	Variable; monitor blood levels and maintain below 20 µg/mL

[a] Anhydrous theophylline equivalent in parentheses.

[b] Administer slowly, no faster than an infusion rate of 25 mg/minute.

Notes

NUTRITIONAL

TABLES

Notes

LISTING OF NUTRITIONAL PRODUCTS FOR INFANTS AND CHILDREN[a]

[a] This section lists, by recommended Therapeutic Uses, nutritional preparations found in the tables that follow (pp. 172 to 196). All preparations are listed by their TRADE NAMES in UPPER CASE TYPE.

169

REGULAR INFANT FORMULAS

TRADE NAME	CAL[a]	CARBOHYDRATE	GRAMS[a]	PROTEIN	GRAMS[a]	FAT	GRAMS[a]	Na[b]	K[b]	Fe[b]
Mature Human Milk	20.1	Lactose	2.13	Human milk	0.31	Human milk	1.15	5.7	17.5	0.02
Whole Cow's Milk	18.6	Lactose	1.43	Cow's milk	1.00	Butterfat	1.02	14.9	46.4	0.01
2% Lowfat Milk	15.2	Lactose	1.46	Cow's milk	1.01	Butterfat	0.59	15.2	47.0	0.01
Skim Milk	10.7	Lactose	1.46	Cow's milk	1.04	Butterfat	0.06	15.8	50.5	0.01
BONAMIL WITH IRON	20.0	Lactose	2.14	Nonfat milk	0.46	Soy oil, coconut oil, soy lecithin	1.08	5.4	18.6	0.15
CARNATION GOOD START	20.0	Lactose, maltodextrin	2.20	Reduced minerals whey	0.48	Palm olein, soy oil, coconut oil, high oleic safflower oil	1.04	4.8	20.0	0.10
ENFAMIL	20.0	Lactose	2.18	Nonfat milk, reduced minerals whey	0.42	Palm olein, soy oil, coconut oil, high oleic sunflower oil	1.06	5.4	21.6	0.14
ENFAMIL WITH IRON	20.0	Lactose	2.18	Nonfat milk, reduced minerals whey	0.42	Palm olein, soy oil, coconut oil, high oleic sunflower oil	1.06	5.4	21.6	0.36
ENFAMIL AR WITH IRON	20.0	Lactose, rice starch, maltodextrin	2.20	Nonfat milk	0.50	Palm olein, soy oil, coconut oil, high oleic sunflower oil	1.02	7.6	21.6	0.36
ENFAMIL 24	24.0	Lactose	2.63	Nonfat milk, reduced minerals whey	0.51	Palm olein, soy oil, coconut oil, sunflower oil	1.27	6.5	25.7	0.17

Product	kcal	Carbohydrate source		Protein source		Fat source				
ENFAMIL 24 WITH IRON	24.0	Lactose	2.63	Nonfat milk, reduced minerals whey	0.51	Palm olein, soy oil, coconut oil, sunflower oil	1.27	6.5	25.7	0.43
GERBER BABY FORMULA WITH IRON	20.0	Lactose	2.13	Nonfat milk	0.45	Palm olein, soy oil, coconut oil, high oleic sunflower oil	1.08	6.6	21.6	0.36
GERBER BABY LOW IRON FORMULA	20.0	Lactose	2.14	Nonfat milk	0.45	Palm olein, soy oil, coconut oil, high oleic sunflower oil	1.08	6.6	21.6	0.01
SIMILAC 20	20.0	Lactose	2.16	Nonfat milk, whey protein concentrate	0.41	High oleic safflower oil, coconut oil, soy oil	1.08	4.8	21.0	0.04
SIMILAC WITH IRON 20	20.0	Lactose	2.14	Nonfat milk, whey protein concentrate	0.41	Hihj oleic safflower oil, cocinut oil, soy oil	1.08	4.8	21.0	0.36
SIMILAC 24	24.0	Lactose	2.50	Nonfat milk	0.65	Soy oil, coconut oil	1.25	8.1	31.4	0.05
SIMILAC WITH IRON 24	24.0	Lactose	2.50	Nonfat milk	0.65	Soy oil, coconut oil	1.25	8.1	31.4	0.42
SIMILAC 27	27.0	Lactose	2.83	Nonfat milk	0.73	Soy oil, coconut oil	1.42	9.1	35.5	0.06
SIMILAC PM 60/40[c]	20.0	Lactose	2.04	Whey protein concentrate, sodium caseinate	0.44	Soy oil, corn oil, coconut oil	1.12	4.8	17.2	0.04

[a] Contents per fluid ounce (liquid) or following standard dilution of powder.
[b] Milligrams per fluid ounce.
[c] Data listed assume standard dilution of powder.

REGULAR FORMULAS FOR TODDLERS

TRADE NAME	CAL[a]	CARBOHYDRATE	GRAMS[a]	PROTEIN	GRAMS[a]	FAT	GRAMS[a]	Na[b]	K[b]	Fe[b]
CARNATION FOLLOW-UP FORMULA	20.0	Corn syrup, maltodextrin	2.64	Nonfat milk	0.52	Palm olein, soy oil, coconut oil, high oleic safflower oil	0.82	7.8	27.0	0.38
NEXT STEP LIQUID	20.0	Corn syrup solids, lactose	2.22	Nonfat milk	0.52	Palm olein, soy oil, coconut oil, high oleic sunflower oil, mono- and diglycerides, soy lecithin	1.0	8.2	26.0	0.36
NEXT STEP POWDER[c]	20.0	Corn syrup solids, lactose	2.22	Nonfat milk	0.52	Palm olein, soy oil, coconut oil, high oleic sunflower oil, mono- and diglycerides, soy lecithin	1.0	8.2	26.0	0.36

[a] Contents per fluid ounce (liquid) or following standard dilution of powder.
[b] Milligrams per fluid ounce.
[c] Data listed assume standard dilution of powder.

174

HYPOALLERGENIC INFANT FORMULAS

TRADE NAME	CAL[a]	CARBOHYDRATE	GRAMS[a]	PROTEIN	GRAMS[a]	FAT	GRAMS[a]	Na[b]	K[b]	Fe[b]
ALIMENTUM	20.0	Sucrose, modified tapioca starch	2.04	Casein hydrolysate, amino acids	0.55	Medium chain triglycerides, safflower oil, soy oil	1.11	8.8	23.6	0.36
GERBER SOY FORMULA	20.0	Corn syrup, sugar	2.01	Soy protein isolate, amino acids	0.60	Palm olein, soy oil, coconut oil, high oleic sunflower oil	1.06	9.4	23.0	0.36
ISOMIL	20.0	Corn syrup, sucrose	2.06	Soy protein isolate, L-methionine	0.49	Soy oil, coconut oil	1.09	8.8	21.6	0.36
ISOMIL DF[c]	20.0	Corn syrup, sucrose	2.02	Soy protein isolate, L-methionine	0.53	Soy oil, coconut oil	1.09	8.8	21.6	0.36
ISOMIL SF[d]	20.0	Hydrolyzed corn starch	2.02	Soy protein isolate, L-methionine	0.53	Soy oil, coconut oil	1.09	8.8	21.6	0.36
LACTO*FREE*	20.0	Corn syrup solids	2.08	Milk protein isolate	0.44	Palm olein, soy oil, coconut oil, high oleic sunflower oil	1.10	6.0	22.0	0.36
NUTRAMIGEN	20.0	Corn syrup solids, modified corn starch	2.20	Casein hydrolysate, amino acids	0.56	Palm olein, soy oil, coconut oil, high oleic sunflower oil	1.00	9.4	22.0	0.36
PREGESTIMIL[e]	20.0	Corn syrup solids, starch, dextrose	2.06	Casein hydrolysate	0.56	Medium chain triglycerides, corn oil, soy oil, high oleic sunflower oil	1.12	7.8	21.8	0.38
PREGESTIMIL 20	20.0	Corn syrup solids, modified corn starch	2.04	Casein hydrolysate	0.56	Medium chain triglycerides, soy oil, high oleic sunflower oil	1.12	9.4	22.0	0.38

TRADE NAME	CAL[a]	CARBOHYDRATE	GRAMS[a]	PROTEIN	GRAMS[a]	FAT	GRAMS[a]	Na[b]	K[b]	Fe[b]
PREGESTIMIL 24	24.0	Corn syrup solids, modified corn starch	2.45	Casein hydrolysate	0.67	Medium chain triglycerides, soy oil, high oleic sunflower oil	1.35	11.3	26.4	0.45
PROSOBEE	20.0	Corn syrup solids	2.12	Soy protein isolate	0.50	Palm olein, soy oil, coconut oil, high oleic sunflower oil	1.06	7.2	24.0	0.36
RCF[f]	20.0		0.00	Soy protein isolate, L-methionine	1.18	Soy oil, coconut oil	2.12	17.4	42.9	0.71
SOYALAC	20.0	Corn syrup, sucrose	2.00	Soybean extract	0.62	Soy oil, linoleic acid	1.10	8.7	23.1	0.30
I-SOYALAC	20.0	Sucrose, tapioca dextrin, potato maltodextrin	2.00	Soybean isolate, amino acids	0.62	Soy oil, linoleic acid	1.10	8.3	23.1	0.38

a Contents per fluid ounce (liquid) or following standard dilution of powder.
b Milligrams per fluid ounce.
c For the dietary management of diarrhea.
d Sucrose-free formula.
e Data assume contents following standard dilution of powder.
f Carbohydrate-free formula.

176

HYPOALLERGENIC FORMULAS FOR TODDLERS

TRADE NAME	CAL[a]	CARBOHYDRATE	GRAMS[a]	PROTEIN	GRAMS[a]	FAT	GRAMS[a]	Na[b]	K[b]	Fe[b]
NEXT STEP SOY LIQUID	20.0	Corn syrup solids, sucrose	2.00	Soy protein isolate	0.60	Palm olein, soy oil, coconut oil, high oleic sunflower oil	1.06	7.2	24.0	0.36
NEXT STEP SOY POWDER[c]	20.0	Corn syrup solids, sucrose	2.36	Soy protein isolate	0.66	Palm olein, soy oil, coconut oil, high oleic sunflower oils	0.88	9.0	30.0	0.36

[a] Contents per fluid ounce (liquid) or following standard dilution of powder.
[b] Milligrams per fluid ounce.
[c] Data listed assume standard dilution of powder.

177

LOW BIRTH-WEIGHT INFANT FORMULAS

TRADE NAME	CAL[a]	CARBOHYDRATE	GRAMS[a]	PROTEIN	GRAMS[a]	FAT	GRAMS[a]	Na[b]	K[b]	Fe[b]
ENFAMIL 22 WITH IRON LIQUID	22.0	Maltodextrins, lactose, citrates	2.35	Nonfat milk, whey protein concentrate	0.62	High oleic sunflower oil, soy oil, coconut oil, medium chain triglycerides	1.16	7.7	23.1	0.40
ENFAMIL 22 WITH IRON[c] POWDER	22.0	Corn syrup solids, lactose	2.35	Nonfat milk, whey protein concentrate	0.62	High oleic sunflower oil, soy oil, coconut oil, medium chain triglycerides	1.16	7.7	23.1	0.40
ENFAMIL PREMATURE 20	20.0	Corn syrup solids, lactose	2.22	Nonfat milk, whey protein concentrate	0.60	Coconut oil, soy oil, mono- & diglycerides, medium chain triglycerides	1.03	7.8	20.6	0.05
ENFAMIL PREMATURE 20 WITH IRON	20.0	Corn syrup solids, lactose	2.22	Nonfat milk, whey protein concentrate	0.60	Coconut oil, soy oil, mono- & diglycerides, medium chain triglycerides	1.03	7.8	20.6	0.36
ENFAMIL PREMATURE 24	24.0	Corn syrup solids, lactose	2.64	Nonfat milk, whey protein concentrate	0.71	Coconut oil, soy oil, mono- & diglycerides, medium chain triglycerides	1.22	9.3	24.5	0.06
ENFAMIL PREMATURE 24 WITH IRON	24.0	Corn syrup solids, lactose	2.66	Nonfat milk, whey protein concentrate	0.71	Coconut oil, soy oil, mono- & diglycerides, medium chain triglycerides	1.22	9.3	24.5	0.36
SIMILAC NATURAL CARE	24.0	Hydrolyzed corn starch, lactose	2.52	Nonfat milk, whey protein concentrate	0.65	Medium chain triglycerides, soy oil, coconut oil	1.29	10.2	30.7	0.09

178

TRADE NAME	CAL[a]	CARBOHYDRATE	GRAMS[a]	PROTEIN	GRAMS[a]	FAT	GRAMS[a]	Na[b]	K[b]	Fe[b]
SIMILAC NEO-CARE[c]	22.0	Corn syrup solids, lactose	2.27	Nonfat milk, whey protein concentrate	0.57	Soy oil, high oleic safflower oil, medium chain triglycerides, coconut oil	1.21	7.3	31.3	0.40
SIMILAC SPECIAL CARE 20	20.0	Hydrolyzed corn starch, lactose	2.12	Nonfat milk, whey protein concentrate	0.54	Medium chain triglycerides, soy oil, coconut oil	1.09	8.6	25.8	0.07
SIMILAC SPECIAL CARE WITH IRON 20	20.0	Hydrolyzed corn starch, lactose	2.12	Nonfat milk, whey protein concentrate	0.54	Medium chain triglycerides, soy oil, coconut oil	1.09	8.6	25.8	0.36
SIMILAC SPECIAL CARE 24	24.0	Hydrolyzed corn starch, lactose	2.52	Nonfat milk, whey protein concentrate	0.65	Medium chain triglycerides, soy oil, coconut oil	1.29	10.2	30.7	0.09
SIMILAC SPECIAL CARE WITH IRON 24	24.0	Hydrolyzed corn starch, lactose	2.52	Nonfat milk, whey protein concentrate	0.65	Medium chain triglycerides, soy oil, coconut oil	1.29	10.2	30.7	0.43

[a] Contents per fluid ounce (liquid) or following standard dilution of powder.
[b] Milligrams per fluid ounce.
[c] Data assume contents following standard dilution of powder.

FORMULAS FOR INFANTS OR CHILDREN WITH SPECIAL METABOLIC DEMANDS

TRADE NAME	CAL[a]	CARBOHYDRATE	GRAMS[a]	PROTEIN	GRAMS[a]	FAT	GRAMS[a]	Na[b]	K[b]	Fe[b]
CALCILO XD[c]	513	Lactose	52.3	Whey protein concentrate, sodium caseinate	11.4	Corn oil, coconut oil	28.7	108	420	9.2
CYCLINEX-1[d]	515	Hydrolyzed corn starch	52.0	Amino acids	7.5	Palm oil, soy oil, hydrogenated coconut oil	27.0	215	760	10.0
CYCLINEX-2[d]	480	Hydrolyzed corn starch	40.0	Amino acids	15.0	Palm oil, soy oil, hydrogenated coconut oil	20.7	1175	1830	17.0
GLUTAREX-1[e]	480	Hydrolyzed corn starch	46.3	Amino acids	15.0	Palm oil, soy oil, hydrogenated coconut oil	23.9	190	675	9.0
GLUTAREX-2[e]	410	Hydrolyzed corn starch	30.0	Amino acids	30.0	Palm oil, soy oil, hydrogenated coconut oil	15.5	880	1370	13.0
HOMINEX-1[f]	480	Hydrolyzed corn starch	46.3	Amino acids	15.0	Palm oil, soy oil, hydrogenated coconut oil	23.9	190	675	9.0
HOMINEX-2[f]	410	Hydrolyzed corn starch	30.0	Amino acids	30.0	Palm oil, soy oil, hydrogenated coconut oil	15.5	880	1370	13.0
I-VALEX-1[g]	480	Hydrolyzed corn starch	46.3	Amino acids	15.0	Palm oil, soy oil, hydrogenated coconut oil	23.9	190	675	9.0

I-VALEX-2[g]	410	Hydrolyzed corn starch	30.0	Amino acids	30.0	Palm oil, soy oil, hydrogenated coconut oil	15.5	880	1370	13.0
KETONEX-1[h]	480	Hydrolyzed corn starch	46.3	Amino acids	15.0	Palm oil, soy oil, hydrogenated coconut oil	23.9	190	675	9.0
KETONEX-2[h]	410	Hydrolyzed corn starch	30.0	Amino acids	3?.0	Palm oil, soy oil, hydrogenated coconut oil	15.5	880	1370	13.0
LOFENALAC[i]	460	Corn syrup solids, modified tapioca starch	59.8	Casein hydrolysate, amino acids	15.2	Corn oil	17.9	216	469	8.6
MEAD JOHNSON PRODUCT 3200 AB[j]	460	Corn syrup solids, modified tapioca starch	60.0	Casein hydrolysate, amino acids	15.0	Corn oil	18.0	220	470	8.7
MEAD JOHNSON PRODUCT 3232A[k]	517	Modified tapioca starch	33.0	Casein hydrolysate	22.0	Medium chain triglycerides, corn oil	33.0	340	860	14.8
MEAD JOHNSON PRODUCT 80056[l]	495	Corn syrup solids, modified tapioca starch	72.0		0.0	Corn oil	23.0	80	340	10.8
MEAD JOHNSON HIST-1 FORMULA[m]	270	Sucrose	17.0	Amino acids	51.0		0.0	1070	2300	34.0
MEAD JOHNSON HIST-2 FORMULA[m]	300	Sucrose	5.4	Amino acids	67.0		0.0	640	1330	15.0
MEAD JOHNSON HOM-1 FORMULA[n]	280	Sucrose	15.9	Amino acids	52.0		0.0	1070	2300	34.0

TRADE NAME	CAL[a]	CARBOHYDRATE	GRAMS[a]	PROTEIN	GRAMS[a]	FAT	GRAMS[a]	Na[b]	K[b]	Fe[b]
MEAD JOHNSON HOM-2 FORMULA[n]	290	Sucrose	3.8	Amino acids	69.0		0.0	640	1330	15.0
MEAD JOHNSON LYS-1 FORMULA[o]	280	Sucrose	21.0	Amino acids	48.0		0.0	1070	2300	34.0
MEAD JOHNSON LYS-2 FORMULA[o]	300	Sucrose	10.5	Amino acids	64.0		0.0	640	1330	15.0
MEAD JOHNSON MSUD-1 FORMULA[h]	280	Sucrose	29.0	Amino acids	41.0		0.0	1070	2300	34.0
MEAD JOHNSON MSUD-2 FORMULA[h]	300	Sucrose	21.5	Amino acids	54.0		0.0	640	1330	15.0
MEAD JOHNSON OS-1 FORMULA[p]	280	Sucrose	27.0	Amino acids	42.0		0.0	1070	2300	34.0
MEAD JOHNSON OS-2 FORMULA[p]	300	Sucrose	18.9	Amino acids	56.0		0.0	640	1330	15.0
MEAD JOHNSON PKU-1 FORMULA[q]	270	Sucrose	17.4	Amino acids	50.0		0.0	1070	2300	34.0
MEAD JOHNSON PKU-2 FORMULA[q]	290	Sucrose	6.2	Amino acids	67.0		0.0	640	1330	15.0
MEAD JOHNSON TYR-1 FORMULA[r,s]	270	Sucrose	21.0	Amino acids	57.0		0.0	1070	2300	34.0

Product									
MEAD JOHNSON TYR-2 FORMULA[f,s]	300	Sucrose	10.7	Amino acids	63.0		0.0	640	1330	15.0
MEAD JOHNSON UCD-1 FORMULA[t]	250	Sucrose	5.8	Amino acids	56.0		0.0	1260	2800	40.0
MEAD JOHNSON UCD-2 FORMULA[t]	290	Sucrose	4.4	Amino acids	67.0		0.0	640	1330	15.0
MSUD DIET[h]	424	Corn syrup solids, modified tapioca starch	63.0	Amino acids	8.1	Corn oil	20.0	184	490	8.9
PHENEX-1[q]	480	Hydrolyzed corn starch	46.3	Amino acids	15.0	Palm oil, soy oil, hydrogenated coconut oil	23.9	190	675	9.0
PHENEX-2[q]	410	Hydrolyzed corn starch	30.0	Amino acids	30.0	Palm oil, soy oil, hydrogenated coconut oil	15.5	880	1370	13.0
PHENYL-FREE[q]	400	Sucrose, corn syrup solids, modified tapioca starch	64.0	Amino acids	19.8	Corn oil, coconut oil	6.6	400	1340	11.9
PRO-PHREE[k]	520	Hydrolyzed corn starch	60.0	Amino acids	Trace	Palm oil, soy oil, hydrogenated coconut oil	31.0	250	825	11.9
PROPIMEX-1[p]	480	Hydrolyzed corn starch	46.3	Amino acids	15.0	Palm oil, soy oil, hydrogenated coconut oil	23.9	190	675	9.0
PROPIMEX-2[p]	410	Hydrolyzed corn starch	30.0	Amino acids	30.0	Palm oil, soy oil, hydrogenated coconut oil	15.5	880	1370	

TRADE NAME	CAL[a]	CARBOHYDRATE	GRAMS[a]	PROTEIN	GRAMS[a]	FAT	GRAMS[a]	Na[b]	K[b]	Fe[b]
PROVIMIN[u]	313		2.0	Casein, amino acids	73.0	Coconut oil	1.4	1200	3300	40
TYREX-2[f]	410	Hydrolyzed corn starch	30.0	Amino acids	30.0	Palm oil, soy oil, hydrogenated coconut oil	15.5	880	1370	13.0
TYROMEX-1	480	Hydrolyzed corn starch	46.3	Amino acids	15.0	Palm oil, soy oil, hydrogenated coconut oil	23.9	190	675	9.0

a Contents per 100 grams of powder. Formula dilution will vary as prescribed by the physician depending on the specific needs of each patient.

b Milligrams per 100 grams of powder.

c Low calcium; vitamin D-free formula for infants with hypercalcemia (as may occur in Williams syndrome) or in osteopetrosis.

d Non-essential amino acid-free formula for infants and toddlers (CYCLINEX-1) or children and adults (CYCLINEX-2) with a defect in a urea cycle enzyme or with gyrate atrophy of the choroid and retina.

e Lysine- and tryptophan-free formula for infants and toddlers (GLUTAREX-1) or children and adults (GLUTAREX-2) with glutaric aciduria type I.

f Methionine-free formula for infants and toddlers (HOMINEX-1) or children and adults (HOMINEX-2) with vitamin B_6-nonresponsive homocystinuria or hypermethioninemia.

g Leucine-free formula for infants and toddlers (I-VALEX-1) or children and adults (I-VALEX-2) with isovaleric acidemia or other disorders of leucine catabolism.

h Branched-chain amino acid-free (isoleucine-, leucine-, and valine-free) formula for infants and toddlers (KETONEX-1, MSUD DIET) or children and adults (KETONEX-2) with branched-chain ketoaciduria (maple syrup urine disease — MSUD).

i Low phenylalanine formula for infants and children with hyperphenylalaninemia including phenylketonuria (PKU).

j Phenylalanine- and tyrosine-free formula for children and adults with disaccharidase deficiencies (lactase, sucrase, and maltase) or impaired glucose transport. It has been used in the management of intractable diarrhea of infancy.

k Protein hydrolysate formula base for children and adults requiring reduced protein intake as in the following conditions: vitamin B_{12} independent methylmalonic acidemia, propionic acidemia, hyperlysinemia, arginosuccinic aciduria, urea cycle disorders, and gyrate atrophy.

l Protein-free formula for infants and toddlers (HIST-1) and children (HIST-2) with histidinemia. B_6-independent form.

m Histidine-free formula for homocystinuria due to cystathionine synthetase deficiency.

n Methionine-free formula for homocystinuria due to lysine ketoglutarate reductase deficiency.

o Lysine-free formula for hyperlysinemia and low threonine formula for infants and toddlers (MEAD JOHNSON OS-1, PROPIMEX-1) or children and adults

p Methionine- and valine-free; low isoleucine and low threonine formula with propionic or methylmalonic acidemia.
(MEAD JOHNSON OS-2, PROPIMEX-2) with propionic or methylmalonic acidemia.

184

q   Phenylalanine-free formula for infants and toddlers (MEAD JOHNSON PKU-1 FORMULA, PHENEX-1) or children and adults (MEAD JOHNSON PKU-2
        FORMULA, PHENEX-2, PHENYL-FREE) with phenylketonuria (PKU) or hyperphenylalaninemia.

r   Phenylalanine- and tyrosine-free formula for children and adults with tyrosinemia type II and type III.

s   Phenylalanine-, tyrosine- and methionine-free formula for infants and toddlers with tyrosinemia type I.

t   Essential amino acids, for hyperammonemia type I, hyperammonemia type II, citrullinemia (arginine to be added), argininosuccinic aciduria (arginine to be
        added), hyperargininemia, hyperornithinemia.

u   Virtually carbohydrate- and fat-free protein base formula used in the preparation of liquid diets for infants and children with chronic diarrhea or other
        malabsorptive disorders that require restriction of fat and carbohydrate intake.

SELECTED SPECIALIZED NUTRITIONAL SUPPLEMENTS AND COMPLETE DIETS

TRADE NAME	CAL[a]	CARBOHYDRATE	GRAMS[a]	PROTEIN	GRAMS[a]	FAT	GRAMS[a]	Na[b]	K[b]	Fe[b]
ADVERA[c]	37.9	Corn maltodextrin, sucrose, soy fiber	6.40	Soy protein hydrolysate, sodium caseinate	1.78	Canola oil, medium chain triglycerides, refined deodorized sardine oil	0.68	31.3	83.8	0.56
ALITRAQ[d]	37.5	Corn maltodextrin, sucrose, fructose	6.16	Soy hydrolysate, whey protein conc., amino acids, lactalbumin hydrolysate	1.98	Medium chain triglycerides, safflower oil	0.58	37.5	45.0	0.55
ENSURE [Liquid][e]	31.3	Corn syrup, sucrose, corn maltodextrin	5.00	Sodium & calcium caseinates, soy protein isolate, whey protein conc.	1.10	High-oleic safflower oil, canola oil, corn oil	0.76	25.0	46.3	0.56
ENSURE [Powder][e]	31.3	Corn syrup, sucrose, corn maltodextrin	4.25	Sodium & calcium caseinates, soy protein isolate	1.13	Corn oil, soy lecithin	1.13	25.0	46.3	0.28
ENSURE BAR[f]	130	High-fructose corn syrup, honey, brown sugar, rice, corn maltodextrin, soy polysaccharide, sucrose, polydextrose, fructose, oat bran	21	Soy protein isolate, whey protein conc., calcium caseinate, nonfat dry milk, whey powder	6	Partially dehydrogenated cottonseed & soy oils, canola oil, high-oleic safflower oil, corn oil	3	115	200	2.7
ENSURE HIGH PROTEIN[g]	28.2	Corn maltodextrin, sucrose	.85	Sodium & calcium caseinates, soy protein isolate	1.50	High-oleic safflower oil, canola oil, soy oil	0.75	36.3	62.5	0.56
ENSURE LIGHT[h]	25.0	Corn maltodextrin, sucrose	4.16	Calcium caseinate	1.25	High-oleic safflower oil, canola oil	0.38	25.0	46.3	0.56

186

Product										
ENSURE PLUS[i]	44.4	Corn maltodextrin, sucrose, corn syrup	5.91	Sodium & calcium caseinates, soy protein isolate	1.63	Corn oil	1.58	31.3	57.5	0.38
ENSURE PLUS HN[j]	44.4	Corn maltodextrin, sucrose	5.91	Sodium & calcium caseinates, soy protein isolate	1.85	Corn oil	1.47	35.0	53.8	0.56
ENSURE PUDDING[k]	50.0	Sucrose, modified food starch	6.80	Nonfat milk	1.40	Partially hydrogenated soybean oil	2.00	48.0	66.0	0.61
ENSURE WITH FIBER[l]	31.3	Corn maltodextrin, sucrose, soy fiber, oat fiber	5.48	Sodium & calcium caseinates, soy protein isolate	1.10	High-oleic safflower oil, canola oil, corn oil	0.76	25.0	46.3	0.56
FORTA DRINK[m]	15.4	Sucrose, pineapple juice solids	2.60	Whey protein conc.	1.00		<0.2	9.0	11.0	0.36
FORTA SHAKE[n]	35.6	Sucrose, lactose	4.38	Milk	2.13	Milk fat	2.00	30.0	101.3	0.56
GLUCERNA[o]	29.6	Corn maltodextrin, soy fiber, fructose	2.85	Sodium & calcium caseinates	1.24	High-oleic safflower oil, canola oil	1.61	27.5	46.3	0.38
INTROLITE[p]	15.6	Maltodextrin	2.08	Sodium & calcium caseinates, soy protein isolate	0.65	Medium chain triglycerides, corn oil, soy oil	0.54	27.4	46.3	0.41
JEVITY[q]	31.3	Corn maltodextrin, corn syrup, soy fiber	4.56	Sodium & calcium caseinates	1.30	High-oleic safflower oil, canola oil, medium chain triglycerides	1.02	27.5	46.3	0.40
JEVITY PLUS[q]	35.6	Corn maltodextrin, corn syrup, fructo-oligosaccharides, oat fiber, soy fiber,	5.14	Sodium & calcium caseinates	1.65	High-oleic safflower oil, canola oil, medium chain triglycerides	1.16	40.0	55.0	0.54
KINDERCAL[r]	31.3	Maltodextrin, sucrose	4.00	Sodium & calcium caseinates, milk protein constituents	1.01	Canola oil, high-oleic sunflower oil, corn oil, medium chain triglycerides	1.33	11.0	38.8	

TRADE NAME	CAL[a]	CARBOHYDRATE	GRAMS[a]	PROTEIN	GRAMS[a]	FAT	GRAMS[a]	Na[b]	K[b]	Fe[b]
NEPRO[s]	59.4	Corn syrup, fructooligo-saccharides	6.60	Magnesium, sodium & calcium caseinates milk protein isolate	2.08	High-oleic safflower oil, canola oil	2.84	25.0	31.3	0.56
OSMOLITE[t]	31.3	Corn maltodextrin	4.45	Sodium & calcium caseinates, soy protein isolate	1.10	High-oleic safflower oil, canola oil, medium chain triglycerides	1.02	18.7	30.0	0.28
OSMOLITE HN[u]	31.3	Corn maltodextrin	4.24	Sodium & calcium caseinates, soy protein isolate	1.31	High-oleic safflower oil, canola oil, medium chain triglycerides	1.02	27.5	46.3	0.40
OSMOLITE HN PLUS[u]	35.6	Corn maltodextrin	4.69	Sodium & calcium caseinates, soy protein isolate	1.31	High-oleic safflower oil, canola oil, medium chain triglycerides	1.02	27.5	46.3	0.40
OXEPA[v]	44.4	Corn maltodextrin, sucrose	3.13	Sodium & calcium caseinates	1.85	Canola oil, medium chain triglycerides, refined deodorized sardine oil, borage oil	2.78	38.8	58.1	0.56
PEDIASURE[w]	29.6	Corn maltodextrin, sucrose	3.25	Sodium caseinate, whey protein conc.	0.89	High-oleic safflower oil, soy oil, medium chain triglycerides	1.47	11.2	38.7	0.41
PEDIASURE WITH FIBER[x]	29.6	Corn maltodextrin, sucrose, soy fiber	3.34	Sodium caseinate, whey protein conc.	0.89	High-oleic safflower oil, soy oil, medium chain triglycerides	1.47	11.2	38.7	0.41
PERATIVE[y]	38.5	Corn maltodextrin	5.25	Partially hydrolyzed sodium caseinate, lactalbumin hydrolysate	1.98	Canola oil, medium chain triglycerides, corn oil	1.10	31.3	51.3	0.46

PORTAGEN[z]	20.0	Corn syrup solids, sucrose	2.30	Sodium caseinate	0.70	Medium chain triglycerides, corn oil, soy lecithin	0.96	11.0	25.0	0.38
PROMOTE[aa]	29.6	Corn maltodextrin	3.85	Sodium & calcium caseinates, soy protein isolate	1.85	High-oleic safflower oil, canola oil, medium chain triglycerides	0.78	30.0	55.8	0.54
PROMOTE WITH FIBER[aa]	29.6	Corn maltodextrin, oat fiber, soy fiber	4.10	Sodium & calcium caseinates, soy protein isolate	1.85	High-oleic safflower oil, canola oil, medium chain triglycerides	0.84	38.8	58.8	0.54
PULMOCARE[bb]	44.4	Corn maltodextrin, sucrose	3.13	Sodium & calcium caseinates	1.85	Canola oil, high-oleic safflower oil, corn oil, medium chain triglycerides	2.76	38.8	58.8	0.56
SUPLENA[cc]	59.4	Corn maltodextrin, sucrose	7.58	Sodium & calcium caseinates	0.89	High-oleic safflower oil, soy oil	2.84	23.1	33.1	0.56
TWOCAL HN[j]	59.4	Corn maltodextrin, sucrose	6.43	Sodium & calcium caseinates	2.47	Corn oil, medium chain triglycerides	2.69	43.1	72.5	0.56
VITAL HIGH NITROGEN[d]	30.0	Corn maltodextrin, sucrose	5.54	Partially hydrolyzed whey, meat & soy, amino acids	1.25	Safflower oil, medium chain triglycerides	0.33	17.0	42.0	0.36
VIVONEX PEDIATRIC[d]	24.0	Maltodextrin, modified starch	3.78	Amino acids	0.72	Medium chain triglycerides, soybean oil	0.71	12.0	36.0	0.30

a   Contents per fluid ounce (liquid) or following standard dilution of powder.
b   Milligrams per fluid ounce.
c   High calorie, high protein, fiber-fortified formula designed for use in adults and children over 4 years old with HIV infection or AIDS.
d   Elemental formula for use in metabolically stressed patients with impaired gastrointestinal function.
e   Complete, balanced nutrition formula for use in adults and children over 4 years old who are on modified diets, at nutrition risk, experiencing involuntary weight loss, recovering from illness or surgery, or on low-residue diets.
f   Complete, balanced nutrition formula for supplemental use with or between meals. Nutritional values listed are per bar.

189

g   High nitrogen formula for use in patients who require additional calories or increased protein needs as in those recovering from surgery or hip fractures and patients at risk of pressure ulcers.

h   Complete, balanced nutrition formula for supplemental use with or between meals. Useful for patients who need lower calorie, low-fat supplementation.

i   High calorie, balanced nutrition formula for use in patients when limited volume is necessary.

j, k High calorie, high nitrogen formula for use in patients with increased calorie and protein needs and when limited volume is necessary.

l   Complete, balanced nutrition formula for use in adults and children over 4 years old. Contents listed are per oz. of pudding.

m   High protein, vitamin-fortified beverage, suitable for use in adults and children over 4 years old who can benefit from increased fiber in the diet.

n   High protein, calcium-rich beverage fortified with vitamins. Data listed assume standard dilution of powder in whole milk.

o   High fiber, low carbohydrate formula for use in adults and children over 4 years old with abnormal glucose tolerance.

p   Half-calorie liquid food used to initiate tube feeding.

q   High protein, high fiber formula for use in adults and children over 4 years old. May be useful in the dietary management of diarrhea and constipation.

r   Isotonic, lactose-free, nutritionally complete formula for use in children 1 to 10 years old with chronic illness, surgery, trauma, or failure to thrive.

s   Moderate protein, low electrolyte, high calorie formula for use in dialyzed adults and children over 4 years old with chronic or acute renal failure.

t   Complete, balanced nutrition formula for use in adults and children over 4 years old sensitive to hyperosmolar feedings. It is also appropriate as an oral feeding for patients experiencing altered taste perception.

u   High protein, complete, balanced nutrition formula for use in adults and children over 4 years old sensitive to hyperosmolar feedings. It is also appropriate as an oral feeding for patients experiencing altered taste perception.

v   Complete balanced nutrition formula for patients with or at risk for acute respiratory distress syndrome.

w   Complete, balanced nutrition formula for use in infants and children over 1 year old.

x   Complete, balanced nutrition formula for use in infants and children over 1 year old who can benefit from increased fiber in the diet.

y   For metabolically stressed patients with injuries such as multiple fractures, wounds, burns, decubitus ulcers, and sepsis.

z   Complete, balanced nutrition formula with medium-chain triglycerides for use where ordinary dietary fats are poorly absorbed.

aa High protein formula for use in patients with pressure ulcers or who are recovering from infection, injury, or surgery; especially for those who are nonambulatory.

bb High fat, low carbohydrate formula for use in adults and children over 4 years old with chronic obstructive pulmonary disease, cystic fibrosis, or respiratory failure.

cc Low protein, nutritionally complete formula designed for the predialyzed patient with acute or chronic renal failure.

ORAL ELECTROLYTE PREPARATIONS

TRADE NAME	SODIUM (mEq/L)	POTASSIUM (mEq/L)	CALCIUM (mEq/L)	MAGNESIUM (mEq/L)	CHLORIDE (mEq/L)	CITRATE (mEq/L)	PHOSPHATE (mEq/L)	OTHER (Gm/L)	CAL/L
BEECH-NUT PEDIATRIC	50	20	0	0	50	29	0	glucose (25)	
INFALYTE	50	25	0	0	45	34	0	rice syrup solids (30)	126
PEDIALYTE[a]	45	20	0	0	35	46	0	dextrose (25)	100
PEDIALYTE FREEZER POPS	45	20	0	0	35	46	0	dextrose (25)	100
PEDIATRIC ELECTROLYTE[a]	45	20	0	0	35	46	0	dextrose (25)	100
REHYDRALYTE	75	20	0	0	65	30	0	dextrose (25)	100
RESOL	50	20	4	4	50	34	5	glucose (20)	84

[a] In Unflavored, Fruit Flavor, or Bubble-Gum Flavor.

191

SELECTED LIQUID VITAMIN PREPARATIONS

TRADE NAME	FORM	UNIT	A IU	D IU	E IU	C mg	B1 mg	B2 mg	B3 mg	B6 mg	B12 µg	Fe mg	F mg	FOLATE mg	Other
POLY-VI-FLOR 0.25 MG	Drop	1 mL	1500	400	5	35	0.5	0.6	8	0.4	2		0.25		
POLY-VI-FLOR 0.25 MG WITH IRON	Drop	1 mL	1500	400	5	35	0.5	0.6	8	0.4	2	10	0.25		
POLY-VI-FLOR 0.5 MG	Drop	1 mL	1500	400	5	35	0.5	0.6	8	0.4	2		0.5		
POLY-VI-FLOR 0.5 MG WITH IRON	Drop	1 mL	1500	400	5	35	0.5	0.6	8	0.4	2	10	0.5		
POLY-VI-SOL	Drop	1 mL	1500	400	5	35	0.5	0.6	8	0.4	2				
POLY-VI-SOL WITH IRON	Drop	1 mL	1500	400	5	35	0.5	0.6	8	0.4		10			
TRI-VI-FLOR 0.25 MG	Drop	1 mL	1500	400	5	35							0.25		
TRI-VI-FLOR 0.25 MG WITH IRON	Drop	1 mL	1500	400	5	35						10	0.25		
TRI-VI-FLOR 0.5 MG	Drop	1 mL	1500	400	5	35							0.5		
TRI-VI-SOL	Drop	1 mL	1500	400	5	35									
TRI-VI-SOL WITH IRON	Drop	1 mL	1500	400	5	35						10			
VI-DAYLIN ADC	Drop	1 mL	1500	400	5	35									
VI-DAYLIN ADC + IRON	Drop	1 mL	1500	400	5	35						10			
VI-DAYLIN MULTIVITAMIN	Drop	1 mL	1500	400	5	35	0.5	0.6	8	0.4	1.5				
VI-DAYLIN MULTIVITAMIN + IRON	Drop	1 mL	1500	400	5	35	0.5	0.6	8	0.4		10			

Product	Form	Volume										
VI-DAYLIN/F ADC	Drop	1 mL	1500	400		35						0.25
VI-DAYLIN/F ADC + IRON	Drop	1 mL	1500	400		35					10	0.25
VI-DAYLIN/F MULTIVITAMIN	Drop	1 mL	1500	400	5	35	0.5	0.6	8	0.4		0.25
VI-DAYLIN/F MULTIVITAMIN + IRON	Drop	1 mL	1500	400	5	35	0.5	0.6	8	0.4	10	0.25
VI-DAYLIN MULTIVITAMIN	Liq	5 mL	2500	400	15	60	1.05	1.2	13.5	1.05	4.5	
VI-DAYLIN MULTIVITAMIN + IRON	Liq	5 mL	2500	400	15	60	1.05	1.2	13.5	1.05	4.5	10

SELECTED TABLET VITAMIN PREPARATIONS

TRADE NAME	FORM	UNIT	A IU	D IU	E IU	C mg	B1 mg	B2 mg	B3 mg	B6 mg	B12 µg	Fe mg	F mg	FOLATE mg	Other
BUGS BUNNY WITH EXTRA C	Chew	1	2500	400	15	250	1.05	1.2	13.5	1.05	4.5			0.3	
BUGS BUNNY PLUS IRON	Chew	1	2500	400	15	60	1.05	1.2	13.5	1.05	4.5	15		0.3	
BUGS BUNNY COMPLETE	Chew	1	5000	400	30	60	1.5	1.7	20	2	6	18		0.4	Pantothenic acid (10 mg), biotin (40 µg), calcium (100 mg), copper (2 mg), phosphorus (100 mg), iodine (150 µg), magnesium (20 mg), zinc (15 mg)
CENTRUM JR. + IRON	Chew	1	5000	400	30	60	1.5	1.7	20	2	6	18		0.4	Pantothenic acid (10 mg), phytonadione (10 µg), biotin (45 µg), calcium (108 mg), copper (2 mg), chromium (20 µg), magnesium (40 mg), phosphorus (50 mg), iodine (150 µg), manganese (1 mg), zinc (15 mg), molybdenum (20 µg)
CENTRUM JR. + EXTRA C	Chew	1	5000	400	30	300	1.5	1.7	20	2	6	18		0.4	Same as CENTRUM JR. + IRON
CENTRUM JR. + EXTRA CALCIUM	Chew	1	5000	400	30	60	1.5	1.7	20	2	6	18		0.4	Calcium (160 mg); others are the same as CENTRUM JR. + IRON
FLINTSTONES	Chew	1	2500	400	15	60	1.05	1.2	13.5	1.05	4.5			0.3	
FLINTSTONES PLUS CALCIUM	Chew	1	2500	400	15	60	1.05	1.2	13.5	1.05	4.5			0.3	Calcium (200 mg)

	Form		Vit A	Vit D	Vit E	Vit C	Thiamin	Riboflavin	Niacin	B6		Iron	Fluoride	B12	Other
FLINTSTONES PLUS EXTRA C	Chew	1	2500	400	15	250	1.05	1.2	13.5	1.05	4.5			0.3	
FLINTSTONES PLUS IRON	Chew	1	2500	400	15	60	1.05	1.2	13.5	1.05	4.5	15		0.3	
FLINTSTONES COMPLETE	Chew	1	5000	400	30	60	1.5	1.7	20	2	6	18		0.4	Pantothenic acid (10 mg), biotin (40 μg), copper (2 mg), calcium (100 mg), phosphorus (100 mg), iodine (150 μg), magnesium (20 mg), zinc (15 mg)
ONE A DAY KIDS COMPLETE	Chew	1	5000	400	30	60	1.5	1.7	20	2	6	18		0.4	Pantothenic acid (10 mg), biotin (40 μg), copper (2 mg), calcium (100 mg), phosphorus (100 mg), iodine (150 μg), magnesium (20 mg), zinc (15 mg)
POLY-VI-FLOR 0.25 MG	Chew	1	2500	400	15	60	1.05	1.2	13.5	1.05	4.5		0.25	0.3	
POLY-VI-FLOR 0.25 MG WITH IRON	Chew	1	2500	400	15	60	1.05	1.2	13.5	1.05	4.5	12	0.25	0.3	Copper (1 mg), zinc (10 mg)
POLY-VI-FLOR 0.5 MG	Chew	1	2500	400	15	60	1.05	1.2	13.5	1.05	4.5		0.5	0.3	
POLY-VI-FLOR 0.5 MG WITH IRON	Chew	1	2500	400	15	60	1.05	1.2	13.5	1.05	4.5	12	0.5	0.3	Copper (1 mg), zinc (10 mg)
POLY-VI-FLOR 1.0 MG	Chew	1	2500	400	15	60	1.05	1.2	13.5	1.05	4.5		1.0	0.3	
POLY-VI-FLOR 1.0 MG WITH IRON	Chew	1	2500	400	15	60	1.05	1.2	13.5	1.05	4.5	12	1.0	0.3	Copper (1 mg), zinc (10 mg)
POLY-VI-SOL	Chew	1	2500	400	15	60	1.05	1.2	13.5	1.05	4.5			0.3	
POLY-VI-SOL WITH IRON	Chew	1	2500	400	15	60	1.05	1.2	13.5	1.05	4.5	12		0.3	Copper (0.8 mg), zinc (8 mg)

TRADE NAME	FORM	UNIT	A IU	D IU	E IU	C mg	B1 mg	B2 mg	B3 mg	B6 mg	B12 µg	Fe mg	F mg	FOLATE mg	Other
SESAME STREET COMPLETE	Chew	1	2750	200	10	40	0.75	0.85	10	0.7	3	10		0.2	Biotin (15 µg), pabtothenic acid (5 mg), calcium (80 mg), iodine (75 µg), magnesium (20 mg), zinc (8 mg), copper (1 mg)
SESAME STREET WITH EXTRA C	Chew	1	2750	200	10	80	0.75	0.85	10	0.7	3	10		0.2	Biotin (15 µg), pabtothenic acid (5 mg), calcium (80 mg), iodine (75 µg), magnesium (20 mg), zinc (8 mg), copper (1 mg)
SUNKIST PLUS EXTRA C	Chew	1	2500	400	15	250	1.1	1.2	13.5	1	5			0.3	Phytonadione (5 µg)
SUNKIST PLUS IRON	Chew	1	2500	400	15	60	1.05	1.2	13.5	1.05	4.5	15		0.3	Phytonadione (5 µg)
SUNKIST COMPLETE	Chew	1	5000	400	30	60	1.5	1.7	20	2	6	18		0.4	Phytonadione (10 µg), biotin (40 µg), pantothenic acid (10 mg), magnesium (20 mg), iodine (150 µg), zinc (10 mg), manganese (1 mg), calcium (100 mg), copper (2 mg), phosphorus (78 mg)
TRI-VI-FLOR 1.0 MG	Chew	1	2500	400		60							1.0		
VI-DAYLIN MULTIVITAMIN	Chew	1	2500	400	15	60	1.05	1.2	13.5	1.05	4.5			0.3	
VI-DAYLIN MULTIVITAMIN + IRON	Chew	1	2500	400	15	60	1.05	1.2	13.5	1.05	4.5	12		0.3	
VI-DAYLIN/F MULTIVITAMIN	Chew	1	2500	400	15	60	1.05	1.2	13.5	1.05	4.5		1.0	0.3	
VI-DAYLIN/F MULTIVITAMIN + IRON	Chew	1	2500	400	15	60	1.05	1.2	13.5	1.05	4.5	12	1.0	0.3	

IMMUNE SERUMS,

VACCINES, and

TOXOIDS

SELECTED IMMUNE SERUMS

GENERIC NAME	COMMON TRADE NAME	PREPARATIONS	COMMON PEDIATRIC DOSAGE
Hepatitis B Immune Globulin (Human)	H-BIG, BAY-HEP B	Inj: 0.5, 1, 5 mL	**Newborns:** 0.5 mL IM within 12 hours of birth. This product is often used in conjunction with Hepatitis B Vaccine.
Immune Globulin (Human)		Inj: 2, 10 mL	**Hepatitis A:** 0.01 mL/lb (0.02 mL/kg) IM. **Measles (Rubeola):** 0.11 mL/lb (0.25 mL/kg) IM. If the child is also immunocompromised, the recommended dose is 0.5 mL/kg (Maximum: 15 mL) IM. **Varicella:** 0.6 - 1.2 mL/kg IM.
Immune Globulin Intravenous (Human)	GAMIMUNE N, 5%	Inj: 0.5 g (10 mL), 2.5 g (50 mL), 5.0 g (100 mL), 12.5 g (250 mL)	**Primary Humoral Immunodeficiency:** 100 - 200 mg/kg (2 - 4 mL/kg) approximately once a month by IV infusion. **Idiopathic Thrombocytopenic Purpura:** Induction: 400 mg/kg by IV infusion (rate = 0.01 to 0.02 mL/kg/min for 30 minutes), daily for 5 days, or 1000 mg/kg by IV infusion for 1 day or 2 consecutive days. **Maintenance:** 400 mg/kg by IV infusion (rate as above.) If an adequate response does not result, the dose can be increased to 800 - 1000 mg/kg by a single IV infusion. May be given intermittently as clinically indicated to maintain a platelet count greater than 30,000/mm^3. **Pediatric HIV Infection:** 400 mg/kg (8 mL/kg) q 28 days by IV infusion.
	GAMIMUNE N, 5% (Solvent/Detergent Treated)	Inj: 0.5 g (10 mL), 2.5 g (50 mL), 5.0 g (100 mL), 12.5 g (250 mL)	
	GAMIMUNE N, 10%	Inj: 1.0 g (10 mL), 5.0 g (50 mL), 10.0 g (100 mL), 20.0 g (200 mL)	
	GAMIMUNE N, 10% (Solvent/Detergent Treated)	Inj: 1.0 g (10 mL), 5.0 g (50 mL), 10.0 g (100 mL), 20.0 g (200 mL)	
	GAMMAGARD S/D, POLYGAM S/D	**Powd for Inj (with diluent):** for a 5% preparation - 2.5 g (50 mL), 5.0 g (100 mL), 10.0 g (200 mL) for a 10% preparation - 2.5 g (25 mL), 5.0 g (48 mL), 10.0 g (96 mL)	**Primary Immunodeficiency Diseases:** 100 mg/kg every month by IV infusion. Initially, patients may receive 200 - 400 mg/kg by IV infusion. The initial recommended infusion rate is 0.5 mL/kg/hr; this may be gradually increased (Maximum: 4 mL/kg/hr for 5% or 8 mL/kg/hr for 10%).

Idiopathic Thrombocytopenic Purpura: 1 g/kg by IV infusion (initial rate = 0.5 mL/kg/hr); may be gradually increased to a maximum of 4 mL/kg/hr for 5% or 8 mL/kg/hr for 10%). The need for additional doses can be determined by response and platelet count. Up to 3 doses may be given on alternate days, if required.

GAMMAR-P I.V.

Powd for Inj (with diluent):
1.0 g (20 mL), 2.5 g (50 mL), 5.0 g (100 mL), 10.0 g (200 mL)

Immunodeficiency Syndrome: 100 - 200 mg/kg q 3 - 4 weeks by IV infusion (rate = 0.01 mL/kg/min, increasing to 0.02 mL/kg/min after 15 - 30 minutes).

SANDOGLOBULIN

Powd for Inj (with diluent):
1 g (33 mL), 3 g (100 mL), 6 g (200 mL)

Immunodeficiency Syndrome: 200 mg/kg every month by IV infusion (rate = 10 - 20 drops (0.5 - 1.0 mL) per min, increasing to 30 - 50 drops (1.5 - 2.5 mL) per min after 15 - 30 minutes). If the clinical response is not adequate, the dose may be increased to 300 mg/kg or the infusion may be repeated more frequently than once a month.

Idiopathic Thrombocytopenic Purpura: 400 mg/kg by IV infusion on 2 - 5 consecutive days (rate as above). If an adequate response does not result, the dose can be increased to 800 - 1000 mg/kg given as a single infusion.

Rabies Immune Globulin
(Human)

IMOGAM RABIES,
BAY-RAB

Inj: 150 units/mL

Should be used in conjunction with Rabies Vaccine. 20 units/kg (0.133 mL/kg) or 9 units/lb (0.06 mL/lb) IM at the time of administration of the first dose of vaccine. If possible, up to half the dose should be used to infiltrate the wound, and the rest administered IM, preferably in a different site from the rabies vaccine, preferably in the gluteal region.

Tetanus Immune Globulin
(Human)

BAY-TET

Inj: 250 units

Routine Prophylaxis:

Under 7 yrs: Dose may be calculated from the body weight (4.0 units/kg IM). However, it may be advisable to administer 250 units IM regardless of the child's size, since theoretically the same amount of toxin will be produced in the child's body as in the adult.

7 yrs and older: 250 units IM.

GENERIC NAME	COMMON TRADE NAME	PREPARATIONS	COMMON PEDIATRIC DOSAGE
Varicella-Zoster Immune Globulin (Human)		**Inj**: 125 units (of varicella-zoster antibody) in 2.0 mL or less	125 units/10 kg (22 lbs) deep IM, up to a maximum of 625 units (5 vials). For patients under 10 kg, administer 125 units (1.25 - 2.0 mL) at a single site; do not give fractional doses. For patients over 10 kg, give no more than 2.5 mL at a single injection site.

SELECTED BACTERIAL VACCINES

GENERIC NAME	COMMON TRADE NAME	PREPARATIONS	COMMON PEDIATRIC DOSAGE
BCG Vaccine, Percutaneous	TICE BCG	Powd for Inj: live culture of BCG bacillus (approximately 50 mg)	Using sterile methods, 1 mL of sterile water for injection, USP (at 4-25 °C) is added to one ampule of vaccine. After vaccine is prepared, the immunizing dose of 0.2 - 0.3 mL is dropped on the cleansed surface of the skin and a percutaneous procedure is followed using sterile multiple-puncture disc applied through the vaccine. The vaccine should flow into the wounds and dry. No dressing is required; keep site dry for 24 hours. Infants under 1 mo: Dosage should be reduced by one-half, by using 2 mL of sterile water when reconstituting. If a vacinated infant remains tuberculin negative to 5TU on skin testing, and if indications for vaccination persist, the infant should receive a full dose after 1 year of age.
Cholera Vaccine		Inj: suspension of killed *Vibrio cholerae* (1.5 and 20 mL vials)	6 mos - 4 yrs: 0.2 mL SC or IM. 5-10 yrs: 0.3 mL SC or IM; or 0.2 mL intradermally. Over 10 yrs: 0.5 mL SC or IM; or 0.2 mL intradermally. Repeat above dose at 1 week to 1 month.
Haemophilus b Conjugate Vaccine	ProHIBiT	Inj: purified capsular polysaccharide (25 μg), conjugated diphtheria toxoid protein (18 μg)/0.5 mL	15 mos - 5 yrs: 0.5 mL IM (one dose).
	PedvaxHIB, Lyophilized	Powd for Inj (with diluent): purified capsular polysaccharide (15 μg), *N. meningitidis* OMPC (250 μg) per dose (0.5 mL) when reconstituted	2-10 mos: 0.5 mL IM (2 doses 2 months apart, with a booster dose at 12 - 15 months). 11-14 mos: 0.5 mL IM (2 doses 2 months apart). 15 mos - 71 mos: 0.5 mL IM (one dose).

[Continued on the next page]

201

GENERIC NAME	COMMON TRADE NAME	PREPARATIONS	COMMON PEDIATRIC DOSAGE
Haemophilus b Conjugate Vaccine [Continued]	PedvaxHIB, Liquid	Inj: purified capsular polysaccharide (7.5 μg), N. meningitidis OMPC (125 μg)/0.5 mL	2-10 mos: 0.5 mL IM (2 doses 2 months apart, with a booster dose at 12 - 15 months). 11-14 mos: 0.5 mL IM (2 doses 2 months apart). 15 mos - 71 mos: 0.5 mL IM (one dose).
	HibTITER	Inj: capsular oligosaccharide (10 μg), diphtheria CRM$_{197}$ protein (approx. 25 μg)/0.5 mL	2-6 mos: 0.5 mL IM (3 doses at 2 month intervals, with a booster dose at 15 months). 7-11 mos: 0.5 mL IM (2 doses 2 months apart, with a booster dose at 15 months). 12-14 mos: 0.5 mL (one dose, with a booster dose at 15 months). 15 mos - 71 mos: 0.5 mL IM (one dose, no booster).
Meningococcal Polysaccharide Vaccine	MENOMUNE-A/C/Y/W-135	Powd for Inj (with diluent): groups A, C, Y, & W-135 combined in a lyophilized powder form	Over 2 yrs: 0.5 mL SC.
Pneumococcal Vaccine, Polyvalent	PNEUMOVAX 23, PNU-IMUNE 23	Inj: purified capsular polysaccharides from 23 most common pneumococcal types (25 μg of each of 23 types)/0.5 mL	Over 2 yrs: 0.5 mL SC or IM.
Typhoid Vaccine		Inj: suspension of heat & phenol inactivated Ty-2 strain of S. typhi organisms (8 units)/mL	Primary immunization: 6 mos - 10 yrs: Two doses of 0.25 mL each, administered SC at an interval of 4 or more weeks. Over 10 yrs: Two doses of 0.5 mL each, administered SC at an interval of 4 or more weeks. Booster doses: 6 mos - 10 yrs: 0.25 mL SC or 0.1 mL intradermally. Over 10 yrs: 0.5 mL SC or 0.1 mL intradermally.

| Typhoid Vi Polysaccharide Vaccine | VIVOTIF BERNA VACCINE | Enteric-Coated Cpsl: 2 - 6 x 10⁹ colony-forming units of viable *S. typhi* Ty21a and 5 - 50 x 10⁹ bacterial cells of non-viable *S. typhi* Ty21a | **Over 6 yrs:** 1 capsule po on alternate days, taken approximately 1 h before a meal with a cold or lukewarm drink, not to exceed body temperature. Complete immunization is the ingestion of 4 capsules as described above. |
| | TYPHIM Vi | **Inj:** purified Vi capsular polysaccharide (25 μg)/0.5 mL | **Primary Immunization (Over 2 yrs):** 0.5 mL IM in the deltoid (adults and children) or the vastus lateralis (children).
Booster doses: 0.5 mL IM q 2 yrs under conditions of repeated or continued exposure. |

GENERIC NAME	COMMON TRADE NAME	PREPARATIONS	COMMON PEDIATRIC DOSAGE
Hepatitis A Vaccine, Inactivated	HAVRIX	Inj (Pediatric Formulation): hepatitis A antigen (360 ELISA units)/0.5 mL	2-18 yrs: Primary immunization of two doses of 0.5 mL IM, given 1 month apart (month 0 and month 1). A booster dose of 0.5 mL is recommended anytime between 6 and 12 months after the primary immunization.
		Inj (Pediatric Formulation): hepatitis A antigen (720 ELISA units)/0.5 mL	2-18 yrs: Primary immunization of one dose of 0.5 mL IM. A booster dose of 0.5 mL is recommended anytime between 6 and 12 months after the primary immunization.
		Inj (Adult Formulation): hepatitis A antigen (1440 ELISA units)/1.0 mL	Adults: Primary immunization of one dose of 1.0 mL IM. A booster dose of 1.0 mL is recommended anytime between 6 and 12 months after the primary immunization.
	VAQTA	Inj (Pediatric/Adolescent Formulation): hepatitis A antigen (25 units)/0.5 mL	2-17 yrs: Primary immunization of one dose of 0.5 mL IM. A booster dose of 0.5 mL should be given anytime between 6 and 12 months after the primary immunization.
		Inj (Adult Formulation): hepatitis A antigen (50 units)/1.0 mL	Adults (over 17 yrs): Primary immunization of one dose of 1.0 mL IM. A booster dose of 1.0 mL should be given anytime between 6 and 12 months after the primary immunization.
Hepatitis B Vaccine (Recombinant)	ENGERIX-B	Inj (Pediatric/Adolescent Formulation): hepatitis B surface antigen (10 µg)/0.5 mL	Birth - 19 yrs: 0.5 mL IM (3 doses: at birth (or at elected date), 1 month later, and 6 months after the first dose).
		Inj (Adolescent/Adult Formulation): hepatitis B surface antigen (20 µg)/1.0 mL	11 yrs - Adult (over 19 yrs): 1.0 mL IM (3 doses: at elected date, 1 month later, and 6 months after the first dose).

RECOMBIVAX HB	Inj (Pediatric Formulation): hepatitis B surface antigen (2.5 µg)/0.5 mL	**Birth - 10 yrs**: 0.5 mL (2.5 µg) SC (3 doses: at birth (or at elected date), 1 month later, and 6 months after the first dose).
	Inj (Adolescent/High Risk Infant): hepatitis B surface antigen (5 µg)/0.5 mL	**11 - 19 yrs**: 0.5 mL (5 µg) SC (3 doses: at the elected date, 1 month later, and 6 months after the first dose).
	Inj (Adult Formulation): hepatitis B surface antigen (10 µg)/1.0 mL	**Over 20 yrs**: 1.0 mL (10 µg) SC (3 doses: at the elected date, 1 month later, and 6 months after the first dose).
Influenza Virus Vaccine (1998-1999 Formula)	**FLUZONE, FLU-SHIELD**	Inj (Subvirion): hemagglutinin antigens of 3 virus strains (A/Beijing/262/95 [H1N1], 15 µg; A/Sydney/05/97 [H3N2], 15 µg; B/Harbin/07/94 (a B/Beijing/184/93-like strain), 15 µg) per 0.5 mL	**6-35 mos**: 0.25 mL IM. (Two doses at least 1 month apart are recommended for children who are receiving the vaccine for the first time. **3-8 yrs**: 0.5 mL IM. (Two doses at least 1 month apart are recommended for children who are receiving the vaccine for the first time. **9-12 yrs**: 0.5 mL IM as a single dose.
	FLUVIRIN	Inj (Purified Surface Antigen): hemagglutinin antigens of 3 virus strains (as listed above) per 0.5 mL	Doses are the same as above.
Japanese Encephalitis Virus Vaccine	**JE-VAX**	Powd for Inj (with diluent): lyophilized virus	**1-3 yrs**: 0.5 mL SC; 3 doses on days 0, 7 and 30. A booster dose of 0.5 mL may be given after 2 years. **Over 3 yrs**: 1 mL SC; 3 doses on days 0, 7 and 30. A booster dose of 1 mL may be given after 2 years.
Measles Virus Vaccine Live	**ATTENUVAX**	Powd for Inj (with diluent): lyophilized attenuated virus	**Over 15 mos**: 0.5 mL SC.
Measles, Mumps, and Rubella Virus Vaccine Live	**M-M-R II**	Powd for Inj (with diluent): lyophilized attenuated Measles and Rubella viruses, lyophilized live Mumps virus	**Over 15 mos**: 0.5 mL SC, preferably into the outer aspect of the upper arm.
Measles and Rubella Virus Vaccine Live	**M-R-VAX II**	Powd for Inj (with diluent): lyophilized attenuated viruses	**Over 15 mos**: 0.5 mL SC, preferably into the outer aspect of the upper arm.

205

GENERIC NAME	COMMON TRADE NAME	PREPARATIONS	COMMON PEDIATRIC DOSAGE
Mumps Virus Vaccine Live	MUMPSVAX	**Powd for Inj (with diluent):** lyophilized live virus	**Over 12 mos:** 0.5 mL SC, preferably into the outer aspect of the upper arm.
Poliovirus Vaccine Inactivated, Trivalent	IPOL	**Inj:** suspension of inactivated poliovirus Types 1, 2 and 3	**Primary Immunization:** Two doses of 0.5 mL SC or IM with an interval of at least 4 weeks, but preferably 8 weeks. The first two doses are usually administered at 2 and 4 mos of age. If a sequential IPV-OPV schedule is used, OPV is recommended to be given at 12 - 18 mos of age and at 4 - 6 yrs of age. The 3rd dose of OPV should follow at least 6 mos but not more than 12 mos after the 2nd IPOL dose. If a full (IPV only) IPOL schedule is used, the 3rd dose of IPOL should be given at 6 - 18 mos of age and at 4 - 6 yrs of age. The 3rd dose should follow at least 2 mos but not more than 12 mos after the 2nd dose. Follow with a 4th dose before entering school at 4 - 6 yrs of age.
Poliovirus Vaccine Live, Oral, Trivalent (Sabin)	ORIMUNE	**Dispette:** attenuated live Sabin strains, Types 1, 2 and 3	**Primary Series:** Administer first dose (0.5 mL po) at approximately 2 months (6 - 12 weeks) of age. The second dose (0.5 mL po) is given not less than 6 and preferably 8 weeks later, commonly at 4 months of age. A third dose (0.5 mL po) should be given at 15 - 18 months of age, but may be given at any time between 12 and 24 months of age. **Older Children and Adolescents (up to 18 yrs):** Unimmunized children and adolescents should receive 2 doses (each 0.5 mL po) given not less than 6 and preferably 8 weeks apart, followed by a third dose (0.5 mL po) 6 - 12 months after the second dose.

Rabies Vaccine	IMOVAX RABIES	**Powd for Inj (with diluent):** freeze-dried suspension of inactivated virus

Supplemental Doses: On entering elementary school, all children who have completed the primary series should be given a single follow-up dose (0.5 mL po). This dose is not required in those who received the third primary dose on or after their 4th birthday.

Pre-Exposure:

Primary Vaccination: Three (3) IM injections of 1.0 mL each: one on Day 0, one on Day 7, and one on either Day 21 or Day 28.

Booster Dose: Not generally used in children.

Post-Exposure: Six (6) IM injections of 1.0 mL each on Days 0, 3, 7, 14, 30, and 90. The first dose should be accompanied by Rabies Immune Globulin or Antirabies Serum. If possible, up to half the dose should be used to infiltrate the wound, and the rest administered IM, in a different site from the rabies vaccine, preferably in the gluteal region.

Post-Exposure of Previously Immunized Persons: Two (2) IM injection of 1.0 mL each; one given immediately, and one given 3 days later.

	IMOVAX RABIES I.D.	**Powd for Inj (with diluent):** freeze-dried suspension of inactivated virus

Primary Vaccination: Three (3) ID injections of 0.1 mL each: one on Day 0, one on Day 7, and one on either Day 21 or Day 28.

Booster Dose: Not generally used in children.

Rubella Virus Vaccine Live	MERUVAX II	**Powd for Inj (with diluent):** lyophilized attenuated virus

Over 12 mos: 0.5 mL SC, preferably into the outer aspect of the upper arm.

Rubella and Mumps Virus Vaccine Live	BIAVAX II	**Powd for Inj (with diluent):** lyophilized attenuated Rubella virus, lyophilized live Mumps virus

Over 12 mos: 0.5 mL SC, preferably into the outer aspect of the upper arm.

GENERIC NAME	COMMON TRADE NAME	PREPARATIONS	COMMON PEDIATRIC DOSAGE
Varicella Virus Vaccine	VARIVAX	**Powd for Inj (with diluent):** live Oka/Merck varicella virus (1350 PFU)	**1-12 yrs:** 0.5 mL SC, preferably into the outer aspect of the upper arm. **13 yrs & over:** 0.5 mL SC and a second 0.5 mL SC dose 4 - 8 weeks later. The outer aspect of the upper arm is the preferred site of injection.
Yellow Fever Vaccine	YF-VAX	**Inj:** over 1×10^5 Plaque Forming Units (PFU) per 0.5 mL	**Over 6 mos:** 0.5 mL SC, preferably into the outer aspect of the upper arm.

SELECTED TOXOIDS

GENERIC NAME	COMMON TRADE NAME	PREPARATIONS	COMMON PEDIATRIC DOSAGE
Diphtheria and Tetanus Toxoids, Adsorbed (DT)		Inj: diphtheria toxoid (15 Lf units), tetanus toxoid (10 Lf units)/0.5 mL Inj: diphtheria toxoid (6.6 Lf units), tetanus toxoid (5 Lf units)/0.5 mL Inj: diphtheria toxoid (12.5 Lf units), tetanus toxoid (5 Lf units)/0.5 mL Inj: diphtheria toxoid (7.5 Lf units), tetanus toxoid (7.5 Lf units)/0.5 mL Inj: diphtheria toxoid (10 Lf units), tetanus toxoid (5 Lf units)/0.5 mL	**Primary Immunization Series:** **Beginning at 6 - 8 weeks of age:** 2 doses (0.5 mL each IM) at an interval of 4 - 8 weeks, followed by a third dose (0.5 mL IM) 6 - 12 months later. When immunization with DT begins in the first year of life (rather than immunization with DTwP), the primary series consists of 3 doses (0.5 mL each), 4 - 8 weeks apart, followed by a fourth dose (0.5 mL) 6 - 12 months after the third dose. **Adults and Children ≥ 7 yrs:** 2 primary doses (0.5 mL each IM) given at intervals of 4 - 8 weeks, followed by a third dose (0.5 mL) 6 to 12 months later.
Diphtheria and Tetanus Toxoids and Whole-Cell Pertussis Vaccine, Adsorbed (DTwP)		Inj: diphtheria toxoid (6.5 Lf units), tetanus toxoid (5 Lf units), pertussis vaccine (est.: 4 protective units)/0.5 mL Inj: diphtheria toxoid (10 Lf units), tetanus toxoid (5.5 Lf units), pertussis vaccine (est.: 4 protective units)/0.5 mL	**Primary Immunization (6 weeks to 6 yrs):** 0.5 mL IM on 3 occasions beginning at 6 weeks of age, then at 4 - 8 week intervals with a reinforcing dose given 1 year after the third injection. **Booster Doses:** 0.5 mL IM when the child is 4 - 6 years old (preferably prior to entering kindergarten or elementary school). However, if the fourth dose of the primary immunization series was administered after the 4th birthday, a booster of DTP prior to school entry is not needed.
	TRI-IMMUNOL	Inj: diphtheria toxoid (12.5 Lf units), tetanus toxoid (5 Lf units), pertussis vaccine (est.: 4 protective units)/0.5 mL	

209

GENERIC NAME	COMMON TRADE NAME	PREPARATIONS	COMMON PEDIATRIC DOSAGE
Diphtheria and Tetanus Toxoids and Acellular Pertussis Vaccine, Adsorbed (DTaP)	ACEL-IMMUNE	Inj: diphtheria toxoid (9 Lf units), tetanus toxoid (5 Lf units), acellular pertussis vaccine (300 hemagglutination units)/0.5 mL	**Primary Immunization (6 wks - 7 yrs):** 3 doses of 0.5 mL each by IM injection. The customary age for the 1st dose is 2 mos, but can be given as young as 6 weeks of age. The recommended dosing interval is 4 - 8 weeks. **Booster Immunization:** A 4th dose is advised at 15 - 20 mos of age. The interval between the 3rd and 4th dose should be at least 6 mos. A 5th dose is recommended at 4 - 6 yrs of age, preferably prior to entrance into kindergarten or elementary school. If the 4th dose was administered on or after the 4th birthday, a 5th dose prior to school entry is not needed.
	TRIPEDIA	Inj: diphtheria toxoid (6.7 Lf units), tetanus toxoid (5 Lf units), pertussis antigens (46.8 μg)/0.5 mL	
	INFANRIX	Inj: diphtheria toxoid (25 Lf units), tetanus toxoid (10 Lf units), pertussis toxin (25 μg), filamentous hemagglutinin (25 μg), pertactin (8 μg)	
Diphtheria and Tetanus Toxoids and Whole-Cell Pertussis and Haemophilus Influenzae Type b Conjugate Vaccines (DTwP-HIB)	TETRAMUNE	Inj: diphtheria toxoid (12.5 Lf units), tetanus toxoid (5 Lf units), pertussis vaccine (est.: 4 protective units), purified Haemophilus b saccharide (10 μg), diphtheria CRM₁₉₇ protein (approx. 25 μg) per 0.5 mL	Beginning at 2 months of age, 3 doses of 0.5 mL IM at approximately 2-month intervals (i.e., at 2, 4, and 6 months of age), followed by a 4th dose (0.5 mL IM) at 15 - 18 mos of age. TETRAMUNE may be substituted for DTP and HibTITER given separately, whenever the recommended schedules for these two vaccines coincide.
Tetanus Toxoid, Adsorbed		Inj: tetanus toxoid (5 Lf units)/0.5 mL	**Primary Immunization:** 0.5 mL IM at 6 - 8 weeks of age, followed by a 2nd dose (0.5 mL) after an interval of 4 - 8 weeks. Give a 3rd dose (0.5 mL) approximately 6 - 12 months after the 2nd dose. **Booster Dose:** 0.5 mL IM every 10 years.
		Inj: tetanus toxoid (10 Lf units)/0.5 mL	
Tetanus Toxoid, Fluid		Inj: tetanus toxoid (4 Lf units)/0.5 mL	**Primary Immunization:** 0.5 mL IM or SC at 6 - 8 weeks of age, followed by a second dose (0.5 mL) after an interval of 4 - 8 weeks, and a third dose (0.5 mL) after another 4 - 8 weeks. Give a fourth dose (0.5 mL) approximately 6 - 12 months after the third dose. **Booster Dose:** 0.5 mL IM or SC every 10 years.
		Inj: tetanus toxoid (5 Lf units)/0.5 mL	

MISCELLANEOUS

TABLES

COMPARISON OF VARIOUS TYPES OF INSULIN

GENERIC NAME	TRADE NAME	SOURCE OF INSULIN (SPECIES)	ONSET OF ACTION (HOURS)	PEAK ACTIVITY (HOURS)	DURATION OF ACTION (HOURS)	HOW SUPPLIED
Insulin Injection (Regular)	REGULAR ILETIN I	Beef and Pork	0.5 - 1	2.5 - 4	6 - 8	Inj: 100 units/mL
	REGULAR ILETIN II	Purified Pork				Inj: 100 units/mL
	REGULAR PURIFIED PORK INSULIN INJECTION	Purified Pork				Inj: 100 units/mL
	HUMULIN R	Human[a]				Inj: 100 units/mL
	NOVOLIN R	Human[a]				Inj: 100 units/mL
	VELOSULIN BR	Human[b]				Inj: 100 units/mL
	NOVOLIN R PENFILL	Human[a]				Inj: 100 units/mL
	NOVOLIN R PREFILLED	Human[a]				Inj: 100 units/mL
Insulin Lispro	HUMALOG	Human[a]	0.25	1 - 1.5	3.5 - 4.5	Inj: 100 units/mL

	Product	Source				Strength
Isophane Insulin Suspension (NPH)	NPH ILETIN I	Beef and Pork	1 - 2	6 - 12	18 - 26	Inj: 100 units/mL
	PORK NPH ILETIN II	Purified Pork				Inj: 100 units/mL
	HUMULIN N	Human[a]				Inj: 100 units/mL
	NOVOLIN N	Human[a]				Inj: 100 units/mL
	NOVOLIN N PENFILL	Human[a]				Inj: 100 units/mL
	NOVOLIN N PREFILLED	Human[a]				Inj: 100 units/mL
Insulin Zinc Suspension (Lente)	LENTE ILETIN I	Beef and Pork	1 - 3	6 - 12	18 - 26	Inj: 100 units/mL
	LENTE ILETIN II	Purified Pork				Inj: 100 units/mL
	HUMULIN L	Human[b]				Inj: 100 units/mL
	NOVOLIN L	Human[a]				Inj: 100 units/mL
Extended Insulin Zinc Suspension (Ultralente)	HUMULIN U	Human[a]	4 - 8	10 - 18	24 - 36	Inj: 100 units/mL

213

GENERIC NAME	TRADE NAME	SOURCE OF INSULIN (SPECIES)	ONSET OF ACTION (HOURS)	PEAK ACTIVITY (HOURS)	DURATION OF ACTION (HOURS)	HOW SUPPLIED
70% Isophane Insulin Suspension + 30% Regular Insulin Injection			0.5	2 - 12	up to 24	
	HUMULIN 70/30	Human[a]				Inj: 100 units/mL
	NOVOLIN 70/30	Human[a]				Inj: 100 units/mL
	NOVOLIN 70/30 PENFILL	Human[a]				Inj: 100 units/mL
	NOVOLIN 70/30 PREFILLED	Human[a]				Inj: 100 units/mL
50% Isophane Insulin Suspension + 50% Regular Insulin Injection			0.5	2 - 5	up to 24	
	HUMULIN 50/50	Human[a]				Inj: 100 units/mL

[a] Produced from bacteria or baker's yeast using recombinant DNA technology.

[b] Produced semi-synthetically by enzymatic conversion of pork insulin.

214

EXOCRINE PANCREATIC ENZYME REPLACEMENTS

TRADE NAME	PRODUCT FORMULATION	LIPASE (Units)	AMYLASE (Units)	PROTEASE (Units)	COMMON PEDIATRIC DOSAGE
COTAZYME	Capsules	8,000	30,000	30,000	1 - 3 capsules po just prior to each meal or snack. Individual cases may require higher dosage and dietary adjustment.
CREON 5	Delayed-Release Capsules (Microspheres)	5,000	16,600	18,750	**Under 6 yrs**: The exact dosage should be selected based on clinical experience for thisage group. Patients can be started on 1 - 2 capsules per meal or snack. Adjust dosage according to the severity of the disease, control of steatorrhea and good nutritional status. Maximum: 6,000 lipase units/kg per meal. **Over 6 yrs**: Initially, 2 - 4 capsules po per meal or snack. Adjust dosage according to the severity of the disease. Maximum: 6,000 lipase units/kg per meal.
CREON 10	Delayed-Release Capsules (Microspheres)	10,000	33,200	37,500	**Under 6 yrs**: Initially, up to 1 capsule po per meal or snack. Adjust dosage according to the severity of the disease. For cystic fibrosis patients, typical doses are 1,500 - 3,000 lipase units/kg/meal po. Adjust dosage according to the severity of the disease, control of steatorrhea and good nutritional status. Maximum: 6,000 lipase units/kg per meal. **Over 6 yrs**: Initially, 1 - 2 capsules po per meal or snack. Adjust dosage according to the severity of the disease. Maximum: 6,000 lipase units/kg per meal.

TRADE NAME	PRODUCT FORMULATION	LIPASE (Units)	AMYLASE (Units)	PROTEASE (Units)	COMMON PEDIATRIC DOSAGE
CREON 20	Capsules (Delayed-Release Microspheres)	20,000	66,400	75,000	**Under 6 yrs:** The exact dosage should be selected based on clinical experience. For cystic fibrosis patients, typical doses are 1,500 - 3,000 lipase units/kg/meal po. Adjust dosage according to the severity of the disease, control of steatorrhea and good nutritional status. Maximum: 6,000 lipase units/kg/meal. **Over 6 yrs:** Initially, 1 capsule po per meal or snack. Adjust dosage according to the severity of the disease. Maximum: 6,000 lipase units/kg per meal.
KU-ZYME HP	Capsules	8,000	30,000	30,000	1 - 3 capsules po taken with each meal or snack. The dosage may be adjusted depending on individual requirements for control of steatorrhea.
PANCREASE	Capsules (Enteric-Coated Microspheres)	4,500	20,000	25,000	1 - 2 capsules po during each meal and 1 capsule with snacks.
PANCREASE MT 4	Capsules (Enteric-Coated Microtablets)	4,000	12,000	12,000	**6 mos - 1 yr:** Children in this age group have responded to 2,000 lipase units/meal po.
PANCREASE MT 10	Capsules (Enteric-Coated Microtablets)	10,000	30,000	30,000	**1 - 6 yrs:** 4,000 - 8,000 lipase units po with each meal and 4,000 lipase units with snacks.
PANCREASE MT 16	Capsules (Enteric-Coated Microtablets)	16,000	48,000	48,000	**7-12 yrs:** 4,000 - 12,000 lipase units po (more if necessary) with each meal and with snacks.
PANCREASE MT 20	Capsules (Enteric-Coated Microtablets)	20,000	56,000	44,000	

Product	Form			Dosage
ULTRASE MT6	Capsules (Enteric-Coated Minitablets)	6,000	19,500	The smallest effective dose should be used. The dosage should be adjusted according to the severity of the exocrine pancreatic insufficiency. Begin with 1 or 2 capsules po with meals and snacks and adjust dosage according to symptoms.
ULTRASE MT12	Capsules (Enteric-Coated Minitablets)	12,000	39,000	
ULTRASE MT18	Capsules (Enteric-Coated Minitablets)	18,000	58,500	
ULTRASE MT20	Capsules (Enteric-Coated Minitablets)	20,000	65,000	
VIOKASE	Powder[a]	16,800	70,000	**Cystic Fibrosis:** 1/4 teaspoonful (0.7 g) po with meals.
	Tablets	8,000	30,000	**Cystic Fibrosis or Chronic Pancreatitis:** 1 - 3 tablets po with meals. **Pancreatectomy or Obstruction of the Pancreatic Ducts:** 1 - 2 tablets po taken q 2 h.
ZYMASE	Capsules (Enteric-Coated Spheres)	12,000	24,000	1 - 2 capsules po with each meal or snack. Individual cases may require higher dosage and dietary adjustment.

a Contents listed are per 1/4 teaspoonful (0.7 g).

217

ANTIDOTES FOR POISONINGS AND DRUG OVERDOSE

ANTIDOTE	EFFECTIVE AGAINST	MECHANISM OF ACTION	RESULT	INITIAL ANTIDOTE DOSE
Acetylcysteine Sodium	Acetaminophen	Biochemical antagonism	Reduced formation of the hepatotoxic metabolite	140 mg/kg po (as a loading dose); maintenance doses of 70 mg/kg are given q 4 h for a total of 17 doses unless an acetaminophen assay at 4 h after ingestion reveals a nontoxic level.
Atropine Sulfate	Organophosphates	Blockade of muscarinic receptors	Decreased cholinergic activity	0.05 mg/kg/dose IV (usual dose is 1 - 5 mg IV) q 4 - 6 h or more frequently prn, until signs of atropine intoxication occur. [Often used in combination with pralidoxime chloride (see below)].
Charcoal, Activated	(Universal)	Adsorption of drugs	Adsorption (inactivation) on the charcoal	1 g/kg po or 15 - 50 g po. First dose may be mixed with 35% - 70% sorbitol solution (in children over 1 year of age) to allow simultaneous administration of a cathartic. May require an NG tube for administration.
Deferoxamine Mesylate	Iron	Chelation	Increased iron excretion	Over 3 yrs: An initial dose of 1.0 g should be administered IV at a rate not to exceed 15 mg/kg/h. This dose may be followed by 500 mg IM q 4 h for 2 doses. Depending on the clinical response, subsequent doses of 500 mg may be administered q 4 - 12 h up to a maximum of 6 g in 24 h. IM is the preferred route for patients not in shock.

218

Drug	Poison	Mechanism	Effect	Dose
Dimercaprol	Arsenic, Mercury, Gold	Chelation	Increased drug excretion	**Mild Arsenic or Gold Poisoning:** 2.5 mg/kg qid by deep IM injection for 2 days, then bid on the 3rd day, and once daily thereafter for 10 days. **Severe Arsenic or Gold Poisoning:** 3 mg/kg q 4 h by deep IM injection for 2 days, then bid on the 3rd day, and twice daily thereafter for 10 days. **Mercury Poisoning:** 5 mg/kg by deep IM injection initially, followed by 2.5 mg/kg once or twice daily for 10 days.
Edetate Calcium Disodium (EDTA)	Lead	Chelation	Increased excretion of lead	Do not exceed 0.5 g/30 lbs (35 mg/kg) bid IM (total, 1.0 g/30 lbs (70 mg/kg) per day). In mild cases, a dose of 50 mg/kg/day should not be exceeded. For young children the total daily dose may be given in divided doses q 8 or 12 h for 3 to 5 days. Repeat, if necessary, in 4 or more days later.
Ethanol (100%)	Ethylene glycol, Methanol	Inhibition of the toxin biotransformation	Reduced formation of toxic products	1 mL/kg in D_5W IV over 15 minutes, then 0.15 mL (125 mg)/kg/h IV. Maintain ethanol levels at ≥ 100 mg/dL.
Ipecac Syrup	(Universal)	Stimulation of the gastric mucosa and chemoreceptor trigger zone	Vomiting	**6 mos - 1 yr:** 5 - 10 mL po, followed by one-half to one glass of water. **1-12 yrs:** 15 mL po, followed by 1 - 2 glasses of water. **Over 12 yrs:** 15 - 30 mL po, followed by 3 - 4 glasses of water. (Repeat the above doses (15 mL) once, in persons over 1 yr, of age, in 20 minutes if vomiting does not occur.)
Methylene Blue	Nitrates, Nitrites	Acts as an electron donor to hemoglobin	Reverse methemoglobinemia	1 - 2 mg/kg IV (of a 1% solution) given over several minutes; dose may be repeated once in 4 h, if necessary.

ANTIDOTE	EFFECTIVE AGAINST	MECHANISM OF ACTION	RESULT	INITIAL ANTIDOTE DOSE
Naloxone Hydrochloride	Opioids	Competitive antagonism at opioid receptors	Displacement of opioids from receptors	0.01 mg/kg IV followed by 0.1 mg/kg IV or IM if needed, in divided doses.
Physostigmine Salicylate	Anticholinergics	Inhibition of cholinesterases	Increased cholinergic activity	0.02 mg/kg IM or by slow IV (not faster than 0.5 mg/min). Dose may be repeated q 5 - 10 minutes until a therapeutic response is obtained or a maximum dose of 2 mg is attained.
Pralidoxime Chloride	Organophosphates and pesticides	Activation of cholinesterase	Decreased cholinergic activity	20 - 40 mg/kg as an IV infusion (in 100 mL of saline, over 15 - 30 minutes). Repeat in 1 h if necessary.
Sodium Thiosulfate	Cyanide	Biotransformation to thiocyanate	Increased renal excretion	7 g/m^2 by slow IV injection (over approximately 10 min). Maximum dose: 12.5 g.
Succimer	Lead	Chelation	Increases excretion of lead	10 mg/kg or 350 mg/m^2 po q 8 h for 5 days; then 10 mg/kg or 350 mg/m^2 po q 12 h for an additional 2 weeks. Repeated courses may be necessary if indicated by weekly monitoring of blood lead concentration. **Approximate dosage by weight: q 8 or 12 h po as described above -** **18-35 lbs (8-15 kg):** 100 mg. **36-55 lbs (16-23 kg):** 200 mg. **56-75 lbs (24-34 kg):** 300 mg. **76-100 lbs (35-44 kg):** 400 mg. **Over 100 lbs (45 kg):** 500 mg.

For address and telephone information of Poison Control Centers throughout the United States, see pages XXX - YYY.

220

POISON CONTROL CENTERS

ALABAMA

Alabama Poison Center, Tuscaloosa
2503 Phoenix Drive
Tuscaloosa, AL 35405
Telephone: (205) 345-0600
            (800) 462-0800 (AL)
Fax: (205) 759-7994

Regional Poison Control Center,
The Children's Hospital of Alabama
1600 Seventh Avenue South
Birmingham, AL 35233-1711
Telephone: (205) 933-4050
            (205) 939-9201
            (800) 292-6678 (AL)
Fax: (205) 939-9245

ALASKA

Anchorage Poison Center,
Providence Hospital
P.O. Box 196604
3200 Providence Drive
Anchorage, AK 99519-6604
Telephone: (907) 261-3193
            (800) 478-3193 (AK)
Fax: (907) 261-3645

Fairbanks Poison Control Center
1650 Cowles Street
Fairbanks, AK 99701
Telephone: (907) 456-7182
Fax: (907) 458-5553

ARIZONA

Arizona Poison and Drug Information Center
Arizona Health Sciences Center
Room 1156
1501 N. Campbell Avenue
Tucson, AZ 85724
Telephone: (520) 626-6016
            (800) 362-0101 (AZ)
Fax: (520) 626-2720

Samaritan Regional Poison Center
Good Samaritan Regional Medical Center
Ancillary-1
1111 East McDowell Road
Phoenix, AZ 85006
Telephone: (602) 253-3334
            (800) 362-0101 (AZ)
Fax: (602) 256-7579

ARKANSAS

Arkansas Poison and Drug Inform. Center,
College of Pharmacy
4301 West Markham Street
Slot 522-2
Little Rock, AR 72205
Telephone: (501) 661-6161
            (800) 376-4766 (AR)

CALIFORNIA

California Poison Control System - Fresno
Valley Children's Hospital
3151 N. Millbrook, IN31
Fresno, CA 93703
Telephone: (209) 445-1222
            (800) 876-4766 (CA)
Fax: (209) 241-6050

California Poison Control System -
  Sacramento
2315 Stockton Boulevard
Sacramento, CA 95817
Telephone: (916) 734-3415
            (800) 876-4766 (CA)
Fax: (916) 734-7796

California Poison Control System - San Diego
University of California at San Diego Medical
  Center
200 West Arbor Drive
San Diego, CA 92103-8925
Telephone: (619) 543-3666
            (800) 876-4766 (CA)
Fax: (619) 692-1867

Los Angeles County Regional Drug & Poison
  Information Center,
LAC & USC Medical Center
1200 North State Street
Los Angeles, CA 90033
Telephone: (213) 226-7741
            (800) 777-6476
Fax: (213) 226-4194

San Francisco Bay Area Regional Poison
  Control Center,
San Francisco General Hospital
Building 80, Room 230
1001 Potrero Avenue
San Francisco, CA 94110
Telephone: (415) 206-5524
            (800) 523-2222
Fax: (415) 821-8513

COLORADO

Rocky Mountain Poison and Drug Center
8802 East 9th Avenue
Denver, CO 80220-6800
Telephone: (303) 629-1123
            (800) 332-3073 (CO)
Fax: (303) 739-1119

CONNECTICUT

Connecticut Regional Poison Center
University of Connecticut Health Center
263 Farmington Avenue
Farmington, CT 06030
Telephone: (203) 679-3473
            (800) 343-2722 (CT)
Fax: (203) 679-1623

DELAWARE

The Poison Control Center
3600 Market Street
Suite 220
Philadelphia, PA 19104
Telephone: (215) 386-2100
Fax: (215) 590-4419

DISTRICT OF COLUMBIA

National Capital Poison Center
3201 New Mexico Avenue, NW
Suite 310
Washington, DC 20016
Telephone: (202) 625-3333
Fax: (202) 362-8377

FLORIDA

**Florida Poison Information Center -
  Jacksonville**
University Medical Center
University of Florida Health Science Center -
  Jacksonville
655 W. 8th Street
Jacksonville, FL 32209
Telephone: (904) 549-4480
            (800) 282-3171 (FL)
Fax: (904) 549-4063

Florida Poison Information Center - Miami
University of Miami
School of Medicine, Department of Pediatrics
P.O. Box 016960 (R-131)
Miami, FL 33101
Telephone: (305) 585-5253
            (800) 282-3171 (FL)
Fax: (305) 242-9762

**The Florida Poison Information Center and
  Toxicology Resource Center**
Tampa General Hospital
P.O. Box 1289
Tampa, FL 33601
Telephone: (813) 253-4444 (Tampa)
            (800) 282-3171 (FL)
Fax: (813) 253-4443

GEORGIA

Georgia Poison Center
Hughes Spalding Children's Hospital
Grady Health System
Box 26066
80 Butler Street, S.E.
Atlanta, GA 30335-3801
Telephone: (404) 616-9000
            (800) 282-5846 (GA)
Fax: (404) 616-6657

Regional Poison Control Center,
Medical Center of Central Georgia
777 Hemlock Street
Macon, GA 31201
Telephone: (912) 633-1427
Fax: (912) 633-5082

IDAHO

Rocky Mountain Poison and Drug Center
8802 East 9th Avenue
Denver, CO 80220-6800
Telephone: (800) 860-0620 (ID)
Fax: (303) 739-1123

ILLINOIS

Illinois Poison Control Center,
Rush-Presbyterian-St. Luke Medical Center
Suite 1900
222 South Riverside Plaza
Chicago, IL 60606
Telephone: (312) 942-5969
(800) 942-5969 (IL)
Fax: (312) 803-5400

INDIANA

Indiana Poison Center
Methodist Hospital of Indiana
I-65 at 21st Street
Indianapolis, IN 46206-1367
Telephone: (317) 929-2323
(800) 382-9097 (IN)
Fax: (317) 929-2337

IOWA

Iowa Poison Center
2720 Stone Park Boulevard
Sioux City, IA 51104
Telephone: (800) 352-2222 (IA)
Fax: (712) 279-7852

KANSAS

Mid-America Poison Control Center,
University of Kansas Medical Center
Room B-400
3901 Rainbow Boulevard
Kansas City, KS 66160-7231
Telephone: (913) 588-6633
(800) 332-6633 (KS)
Fax: (913) 588-2350

Stormont-Vail Regional Medical Center
Emergency Department
1500 S.W. 10th
Topeka, KS 66604-1353
Telephone: (913) 354-6100
Fax: (913) 354-5004

KENTUCKY

Kentucky Regional Poison Center
Suite 572, Medical Towers S.
234 E. Gray Street
Louisville, KY 40202
Telephone: (502) 589-8222
Fax: (502) 629-7277

LOUISIANNA

Louisianna Drug & Poison Information Center
Northeast Louisianna University
Sugar Hall
Monroe, LA 72109-6430
Telephone: (318) 342-1710
(800) 256-9822 (LA)
Fax: (318) 342-1744

MAINE

Maine Poison Center
Maine Medical Center
22 Bramhall Street
Portland, ME 04102
Telephone: (207) 871-2950
(800) 442-6305 (ME)
Fax: (207) 871-6226

MARYLAND

Maryland Poison Center
20 North Pine Street
Baltimore, MD 21201
Telephone: (410) 528-7701
(800) 492-2414 (MD)
Fax: (410) 706-7184

MASSACHUSETTS

Massachusetts Poison Control System
300 Longwood Avenue
Boston, MA 02115
Telephone: (617) 232-2120
(800) 682-9211 (MA)
Fax: (617) 738-0032

MICHIGAN

Poison Control Center
Children's Hospital of Michigan
4160 John Road
Harper Office Building, Suite 616
Detroit, MI 48201
Telephone: (313) 745-5711
(800) 764-7661 (MI)
Fax: (313) 745-5493

Spectrum Health Regional Poison Center
1840 Wealthy SE
Grand Rapids, MI 49506-2968
Telephone: (616) 774-5329
(800) 764-7661 (MI)
Fax: (616) 774-7204

MINNESOTA

Hennepin Regional Poison Center
Hennepin County Medical Center
701 Park Avenue South
Minneapolis, MN 55415
Telephone: (612) 347-3141
(800) 764-7661 (MN)
Fax: (612) 904-4289

Minnesota Regional Poison Center
8100 34th Avenue, South
P.O. Box 1309
Minneapolis, MN 55440-1309
Telephone: (612) 221-2113
(800) 222-1222 (MN)
Fax: (612) 851-8166

MISSISSIPPI

Mississippi Regional Poison Control
University of Mississippi Medical Center
2500 North State Street
Jackson, MS 39216
Telephone: (601) 354-7660
Fax: (601) 984-1676

Poison Center
Forrest General Hospital
400 South 28th Avenue
Hattiesburg, MS 39401
Telephone: (601) 288-2100

MISSOURI

Cardinal Glennon Children's Hospital
  Regional Poison Center
1465 S. Grand Boulevard
St. Louis, MO 63104
Telephone: (314) 772-5200
(800) 366-8888 (MO)
Fax: (314) 577-5355

Poison Control Center
Children's Mercy Hospital
2401 Gillham Road
Kansas City, MO 64108
Telephone: (816) 234-3430
Fax: (816) 234-3421

MONTANA

Rocky Mountain Poison and Drug Center
8802 East 9th Avenue
Denver, CO 80220-6800
Telephone: (800) 525-5042 (MT)
Fax: (303) 739-1119

NEBRASKA

The Poison Center
8301 Dodge Street
Omaha, NE 68114
Telephone: (402) 390-5555 (Omaha)
(800) 955-9119 (NE)

NEVADA

Rocky Mountain Poison and Drug Center
8802 East 9th Avenue
Denver, CO 80220-6800
Telephone: (303) 629-1123
(800) 446-1123 (NV)
Fax: (303) 739-1119

Poison Center,
Washoe Medical Center
77 Pringle Way
Reno, NV 89520
Telephone: (702) 328-4129
Fax: (702) 328-5555

NEW HAMPSHIRE

New Hampshire Poison Information Center,
Dartmouth-Hitchcock Medical Center
1 Medical Center Drive
Lebanon, NH 03756
Telephone: (603) 650-5000
(800) 562-8236 (NH)
Fax: (603) 650-8986

NEW JERSEY

New Jersey Poison Information and
Education System
201 Lyons Avenue
Newark, NJ 07112
Telephone: (800) 764-7661 (NJ)
Fax: (201) 705-8098

Warren Hospital
Poison Control Center
185 Roseberry Street
Phillipsburg, NJ 08865
Telephone: (908) 859-6767
(800) 962-1253 (NJ)
Fax: (908) 859-6812

NEW MEXICO

New Mexico Poison and Drug Information
Center
University of New Mexico
Health Sciences Library, Room 125
Albuquerque, NM 87131-1076
Telephone: (505) 843-2551
(800) 432-6866 (NM)
Fax: (505) 277-5892

NEW YORK

Central New York Poison Control Center
SUNY Health Science Center
750 East Adams Street
Syracuse, NY 13203
Telephone: (315) 476-4766
(800) 252-5665 (NY)
Fax: (315) 464-7077

Finger Lakes Regional Poison Center
University of Rochester Medical Center
601 Elmwood Avenue
Box 321, Room G-3275
Rochester, NY 14642
Telephone: (716) 275-3232
(800) 333-0542 (NY)
Fax: (716) 244-1677

Hudson Valley Regional Poison Center
Phelps Memorial Hospital Center
701 N. Broadway
Sleepy Hollow, NY 10590
Telephone: (914) 366-3030
(800) 336-6997 (NY)
Fax: (914) 353-1050

Long Island Regional Poison Control Center
Winthrop University Hospital
259 First Street
Mineola, NY 11501
Telephone: (516) 542-2323
Fax: (516) 739-2070

New York City Poison Control Center
New York City Department of Health
455 First Avenue, Room 123
New York, NY 10016
Telephone: (212) 340-4494
(212) POISONS
[764-7667]
Fax: (212) 447-8223

Western New York Regional Poison Control
Center
Children's Hospital of Buffalo
219 Bryant Street
Buffalo, NY 14222
Telephone: (716) 878-7654
(800) 888-7655 (NY &
Western PA)

NORTH CAROLINA

Carolinas Poison Center
Carolinas Medical Center
5000 Airport Center Parkway
Suite B
P.O. Box 32861
Charlotte, NC 28232
Telephone: (704) 355-4000
(800) 848-6946 (NC)

Western North Carolina Poison Control
Center,
Memorial Mission Hospital
509 Biltmore Avenue
Asheville, NC 28801
Telephone: (704) 255-4490
(800) 542-4225 (NC)
Fax: (704) 255-4467

NORTH DAKOTA

North Dakota Poison Information Center,
Meritcare Medical Center
720 North 4th Street
Fargo, ND 58122
Telephone: (701) 234-5575
(800) 732-2200 (ND)
Fax: (701) 234-5090

OHIO

Central Ohio Poison Center
Columbus Children's Hospital
700 Children's Drive
Columbus, OH 43205-2696
Telephone: (614) 228-1323
(800) 682-7625 (OH)
Fax: (614) 221-2672

Cincinnati Drug & Poison Information Center
and Regional Poison Control System
2368 Victory Parkway
Suiye 300
Cincinnati, OH 45206
Telephone: (513) 558-5111
(800) 872-5111 (OH)
Fax: (513) 558-5301

Greater Cleveland Poison Control Center
11100 Euclid Avenue
Cleveland, OH 44106
Telephone: (216) 231-4455
(888) 231-4455
Fax: (216) 844-3242

Greater Dayton Area Hospital Association
Central Ohio Poison Center
700 Children's Drive
Columbus, OH 43205-2696
Telephone: (513) 222-2227
(800) 762-0727 (OH)

Poison Information Center of NW Ohio,
Medical College of Ohio Hospital
3000 Arlington Avenue
Toledo, OH 43614
Telephone: (419) 381-3897
(800) 589-3897 (OH)
Fax: (419) 381-6066

OKLAHOMA

Oklahoma Poison Control Center,
University of Oklahoma and Children's
Hospital of Oklahoma
940 Northeast 13th Street
Oklahoma City, OK 73104
Telephone: (405) 271-5454
(800) 522-4611 (OK)
Fax: (405) 271-1816

OREGON

Oregon Poison Center
Oregon Health Sciences University
3181 S.W. Sam Jackson Park Road
Portland, OR 97201
Telephone: (503) 494-8968
(800) 452-7165 (OR)
Fax: (503) 494-4980

PENNSYLVANIA

Central Pennsylvania Poison Center
University Hospital, Milton S. Hershey
   Medical Center
Hershey, PA 17033
Telephone: (717) 531-6111
             (800) 521-6110 (PA)
Fax: (717) 531-6932

Pittsburgh Poison Center
3705 Fifth Avenue
Pittsburgh, PA 15213
Telephone: (412) 681-6669
Fax: (412) 692-7497

The Poison Control Center
3600 Market Street, Suite 220
Philadelphia, PA 19104-2641
Telephone: (215) 386-2100
             (800) 722-7112 (PA)
Fax: (215) 590-4419

RHODE ISLAND

Lifespan Poison Center
Rhode Island Hospital
593 Eddy Street
Providence, RI 02903
Telephone: (401) 277-5727
Fax: (401) 444-8062

SOUTH CAROLINA

Palmetto Poison Center,
College of Pharmacy,
University of South Carolina
Columbus, SC 29208
Telephone: (803) 777-1117
             (800) 922-1117 (SC)
Fax: (803) 777-6127

SOUTH DAKOTA

Poison Control Center,
St. Luke's Midland Regional Medical Center
305 South State Street
Aberdeen, SD 57401
Telephone: (605) 622-5100
             (800) 592-1889

TENNESSEE

Middle Tennessee Poison Center
The Center for Clinical Toxicology
Vanderbilt University Medical Center
1161 21st Avenue, South
501 Oxford House
Nashville, TN 37232-4632
Telephone: (615) 936-2034
             (800) 288-9999 (TN)
Fax: (615) 936-2046

Southern Poison Center
875 Monroe Avenue
Suite 104
Memphis, TN 38163
Telephone: (901) 528-6048
             (800) 288-9999 (TN)
Fax: (901) 448-5419

TEXAS

Central Texas Poison Center
Scott & White Memorial Hospital
2401 South 31th Street
Temple, TX 76508-2780
Telephone: (254) 724-7401
             (800) 764-7661 (TX)
Fax: (254) 724-1731

North Texas Poison Center
P.O. Box 35926
5201 Harry Hines Boulevard
Dallas, TX 75235
Telephone: (214) 590-6625
             (800) 764-7661 (TX)
Fax: (214) 590-5008

Southeast Texas Poison Center
The University of Texas Medical Branch
301 University Avenue
Galveston, TX 77550-2780
Telephone: (409) 765-1420
             (800) 764-7661 (TX)
Fax: (409) 772-3917

UTAH

Utah Poison Control Center
410 Chipeta Way
Suite 230
Salt Lake City, UT 84108
Telephone: (801) 581-2151
(800) 456-7707 (UT)
Fax: (801) 581-4199

VERMONT

Vermont Poison Center
Fletcher Allen Health Care
111 Colchester Avenue
Burlington, VT 05401
Telephone: (802) 658-3456
Fax: (802) 656-4802

VIRGINIA

Blue Ridge Pison Center
Blue Ridge University of Virginia
 Medical Center
P.O. Box 437
Charlottesville, VA 22908
Telephone: (804) 924-5543
(800) 451-1428 (VA)
Fax: (804) 971-8657

Virginia Poison Center,
Virginia Commonwealth University
P.O. Box 980522
Richmond, VA 23298-0522
Telephone: (804) 828-9123
Fax: (804) 828-5291

WASHINGTON

Washington Poison Center
155 N.E. 100th Street
Suite 400
Seattle, WA 98125-8012
Telephone: (206) 526-2121
(800) 732-6985 (WA)
Fax: (206) 526-8490

WEST VIRGINIA

West Virginia Poison Center
3110 MacCorkle Avenue, S.E.
Charleston, WV 25304
Telephone: (304) 348-4211
(800) 642-3625 (WV)
Fax: (304) 348-9560

WISCOSIN

Children's Hospital Poison Center
Children's Hospital of Wiscosin
9000 W. Wisconsin Avenue
P.O. Box 1997
Milwaukee, WI 53201
Telephone: (414) 266-2222
(800) 815-8855 (WI)
Fax: (414) 266-2820

Poison Control Center,
University of Wiscosin Hospital and Clinics
600 Highland Avenue
F6-133
Madison, WI 53792
Telephone: (608) 262-3702
(800) 815-8855 (WI)

WYOMING

The Poison Center
8301 Dodge Street
Omaha, NE 68114
Telephone: (402) 390-5555 (Omaha)
(800) 955-9119 (WY)

SELECTED SUGAR-FREE, DYE-FREE AND ALCOHOL-FREE PREPARATIONS

TRADE NAME	THERAPEUTIC CATEGORY	PAGE NO.	SUGAR FREE	DYE FREE	ALCOHOL FREE
BENADRYL ALLERGY Liquid	Antihistamine	52			X
BENADRYL DYE-FREE Liquid	Antihistamine	52	X	X	X
BENADRYL DYE-FREE Soft-Gel Capsules	Antihistamine	52		X	
BUGS BUNNY PLUS IRON Chewable Tablets	Multiple Vitamin	194	X		
BUGS BUNNY WITH EXTRA C Chewable Tablets	Multiple Vitamin	194	X		
BUGS BUNNY COMPLETE Tablets	Multiple Vitamin	194	X		
CEROSE-DM Liquid	Decongestant-Antihistamine-Antitussive	120	X		
DECONAMINE Syrup	Decongestant-Antihistamine	123		X	X
DELSYM Syrup	Antitussive	49			X
DEMEROL Syrup (C-II)	Opioid Analgesic	75			X
DIMETAPP Elixir	Decongestant-Antihistamine	124			X
DIMETAPP DM Elixir	Decongestant-Antihistamine-Antitussive	124			X
DRIXORAL Syrup	Decongestant-Antihistamine	125			X
ELIXOPHYLLIN Capsules	Bronchodilator	101		X	
ELIXOPHYLLIN GG Liquid	Antiasthmatic	126	X	X	X
FEDAHIST EXPECTORANT Syrup	Decongestant-Expectorant	127	X		X

229

TRADE NAME	THERAPEUTIC CATEGORY	PAGE NO.	SUGAR FREE	DYE FREE	ALCOHOL FREE
HALEY'S M-O Liquid	Laxative	128	X		
ISOMIL SF	Infant Formula	175	X		
KAOPECTATE Caplets	Antidiarrheal	28			X
KAOPECTATE Liquid	Antidiarrheal	28			X
KONSYL Powder	Bulk Laxative	93	X		
MARAX Tablets	Antiasthmatic	129		X	
MARAX-DF Syrup	Antiasthmatic	129		X	
NALDECON-DX PEDIATRIC Solution (Drops)	Decongestant-Expectorant-Antitussive	131	X		X
NALDECON-EX CHILDREN'S Syrup	Decongestant-Expectorant	131	X		X
NALDECON-EX PEDIATRIC Solution (Drops)	Decongestant-Expectorant	131	X		X
PEDIACARE ALLERGY FORMULA Liquid	Antihistamine	39			X
PEDIAPRED Liquid	Corticosteroid	89	X	X	X
PEPTO-BISMOL Chewable Tablets	Antidiarrheal	32	X		
PEPTO-BISMOL Suspension	Antidiarrheal	32	X		
PEPTO-BISMOL MAXIMUM STRENGTH Suspension	Antidiarrheal	32	X		
PERDIEM Granules	Bulk Laxative-Irritant Laxative	135		X	
ROBITUSSIN Syrup	Expectorant	64			X

Product	Category	Page			
RONDEC Syrup	Decongestant-Antihistamine	140	X		X
RYNA Liquid	Decongestant-Antihistamine	141	X	X	X
RYNA-C Liquid	Antitussive-Decongestant-Antihistamine	141	X	X	X
RYNA-CX Liquid (C-V)	Antitussive-Decongestant	141	X	X	X
SLO-BID Extended-Release Capsules	Bronchodilator	101		X	
SLO-PHYLLIN Syrup	Bronchodilator	101	X		X
SLO-PHYLLIN Tablets	Bronchodilator	101		X	
SLO-PHYLLIN GG Syrup	Antiasthmatic	143		X	X
TEMPRA QUICKLETS Chewable Tablets (Children's Strength)	Non-Opioid Analgesic, Antipyretic	20			X
TEMPRA QUICKLETS Chewable Tablets (Junior Strength)	Non-Opioid Analgesic, Antipyretic	20			X
THEO-DUR Extended-Release Tablets	Bronchodilator	101		X	
THEOLAIR Liquid	Bronchodilator	102			X
TRIAMINIC AM COUGH AND DECONGESTANT FORMULA Liquid	Decongestant-Antitussive	145		X	X
TRIAMINIC-DM Syrup	Decongestant-Antitussive	145			X
TRIAMINIC NIGHT TIME Liquid	Decongestant-Antihistamine-Antitussive	146			X
TRIAMINIC SORE THROAT FORMULA Liquid	Decongestant-Antitussive-Analgesic	146			X
TRIAMINIC Syrup	Decongestant-Antihistamine	147			X

TRADE NAME	THERAPEUTIC CATEGORY	PAGE NO.	SUGAR FREE	DYE FREE	ALCOHOL FREE
TRIAMINICOL MULTI-SYMPTOM RELIEF Syrup	Decongestant-Antihistamine-Antitussive	147			×
TUSSAR-DM Liquid	Decongestant-Antihistamine-Antitussive	147			×
TUSSI-ORGANIDIN NR Liquid (C-V)	Antitussive-Expectorant	148	×		×
TUSSI-ORGANIDIN DM NR Liquid	Antitussive-Expectorant	148	×		×
TYLENOL, INFANTS' Solution (Drops)	Non-Opioid Analgesic, Antipyretic	20			×
TYLENOL, CHILDREN'S Elixir	Non-Opioid Analgesic, Antipyretic	20			×
TYLENOL, CHILDREN'S Chewable Tablets	Non-Opioid Analgesic, Antipyretic	20			×
TYLENOL COLD, CHILDREN'S, Liquid	Analgesic-Antihistamine-Decongestant	148			×
VICKS 44e, PEDIATRIC Liquid	Antitussive-Expectorant	151			×
VICKS 44m COUGH & COLD RELIEF, PEDIATRIC Liquid	Antitussive-Decongestant-Antihistamine	151			×
VI-DAYLIN ADC Drops	Multiple Vitamin	192	×		
VI-DAYLIN ADC + IRON Drops	Multiple Vitamin	192	×		
VI-DAYLIN MULTIVITAMIN Drops	Multiple Vitamin	192	×		
VI-DAYLIN MULTIVITAMIN + IRON Drops	Multiple Vitamin	192	×		
VI-DAYLIN/F ADC Drops	Multiple Vitamin	193	×		

VI-DAYLIN/F ADC + IRON Drops	Multiple Vitamin	193	X
VI-DAYLIN/F MULTIVITAMIN Drops	Multiple Vitamin	193	X
VI-DAYLIN/F MULTIVITAMIN + IRON Drops	Multiple Vitamin	193	X

(C-II): Controlled Substance, Schedule II
(C-V): Controlled Substance, Schedule V

Notes

GROWTH CHARTS

The following eight growth charts (pp. 236 - 243) were kindly provided as a service of Ross Laboratories, Columbus, Ohio; all were adapted from: Hamill, P.V.V., T.A. Drizd, C.L. Johnson, R.B. Reed, A.F. Roche, and W.M. Moore: "Physical Growth: National Center for Health Statistics Percentiles", *Am. J. Clin. Nutr.* **32**: 607-629, 1979.

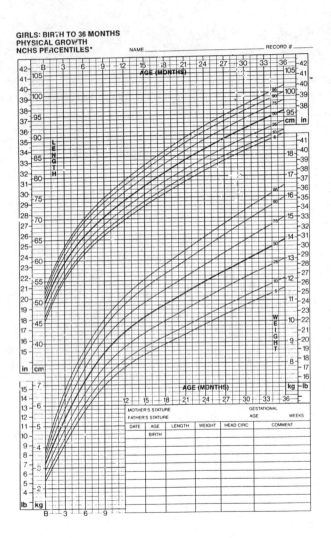

GIRLS: BIRTH TO 36 MONTHS
PHYSICAL GROWTH
NCHS PERCENTILES*

NAME _____ RECORD # _____

236

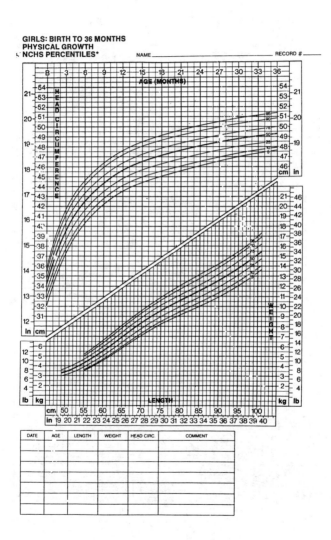

GIRLS: BIRTH TO 36 MONTHS
PHYSICAL GROWTH
NCHS PERCENTILES*

GIRLS: 2 TO 18 YEARS
PHYSICAL GROWTH
NCHS PERCENTILES*

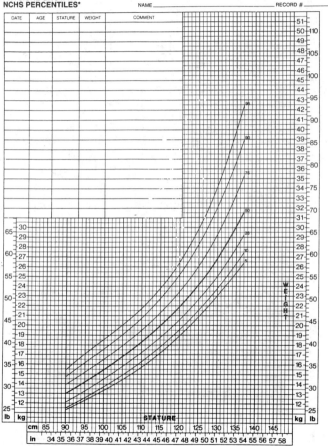

GIRLS: PREPUBESCENT
PHYSICAL GROWTH
NCHS PERCENTILES*

NAME _____ RECORD # _____

DATE	AGE	STATURE	WEIGHT	COMMENT

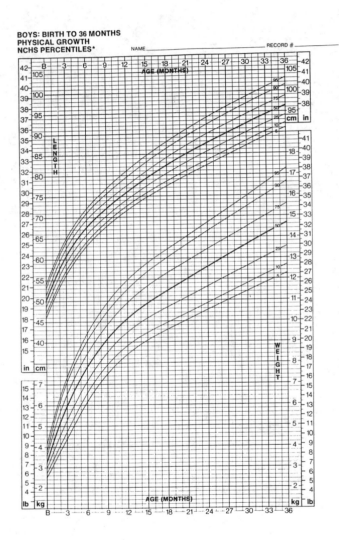

240

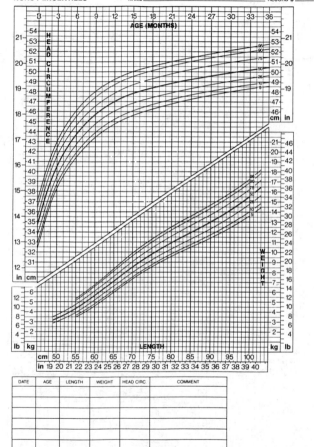

DATE	AGE	LENGTH	WEIGHT	HEAD CIRC	COMMENT

241

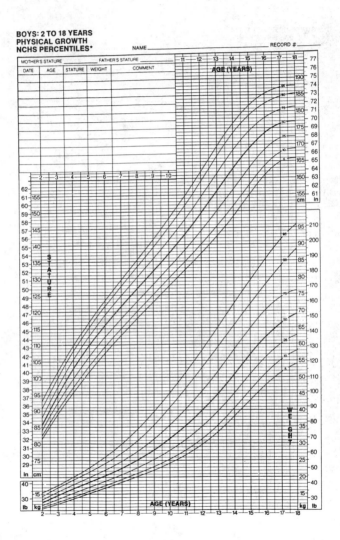

BOYS: 2 TO 18 YEARS
PHYSICAL GROWTH
NCHS PERCENTILES*

NAME_____   RECORD #_____

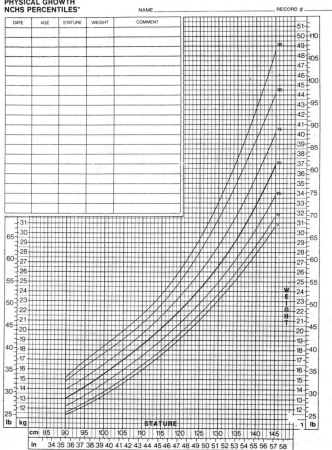

DATE	AGE	STATURE	WEIGHT	COMMENT

Notes

PRESCRIPTION WRITING

INTRODUCTION

A **prescription** is an order for a specific medication for a specified patient at a particular time. It is the way in which a physician (or another health care professional) communicates a patient's selected drug therapy to the pharmacist and instructs the patient on how to use the prescribed medication. The prescription order may be given by a physician, dentist, veterinarian, physician assistant, nurse practitioner, or any other legally-recognized medical practitioner; the order may be written and signed or it may be oral, in which case the pharmacist is required to transcribe it into written form and obtain the prescriber's signature, if necessary, at a later time.

The transfer of the therapeutic information from prescriber to pharmacist to patient must be clear. With all of the many drug products available to the prescriber, it is easy to understand how drug strengths, dosage forms, and dosage regimens can be confused. Many drug names may also look alike (especially when written hastily) or may sound alike (when garbled over the telephone). Furthermore, numerous studies have indicated that 25% to 50% of patients do not use their prescription medication properly; the patient often fails to take the drug or uses the medication either in an incorrect dose, at an improper time, or for the wrong condition. Most errors can be traced to the prescription order or the failure of the prescriber to adequately communicate this information to the patient.

In order that these types of errors be avoided and the patient gain the maximum benefit from the prescribed drugs, it is important for the prescriber to understand the basic principles of prescription writing.

COMPOSITION OF THE PRESCRIPTION ORDER

A complete prescription order is composed of eight parts and follows a standardized format which facilitates its interpretation by the pharmacist. The eight major parts of a prescription order include:

1. The date prescribed
2. The name, address, and age of the patient
3. The superscription
4. The inscription
5. The subscription
6. The signa
7. The renewal information
8. The name of the prescriber

Figure 1 illustrates a sample precompounded prescription order with the eight major elements numbered for reference purposes.

1. **The Date Prescribed** - The date on which a prescription was issued is important since a patient may not always have a prescription filled on the day it was written; days, weeks, months, or on occasion, years may pass before a patient presents the prescription to the pharmacist. Medications are intended for a patient at a particular time; the date prescribed may reveal that the presented prescription was not filled when written and now, for example, months later, the patient has symptoms which are exactly the same as the last time" and is attempting to self-diagnose and self-medicate. Furthermore, drugs controlled by special laws and regulations, e.g., the Controlled Substances Act of 1970, cannot be dispensed or renewed more than six months from the date prescribed. Therefore, the date prescribed provides an accurate record of when a prescription was originally issued to the patient.

TELEPHONE (215) 555-2474

John V. Smith, M.D.
Paula A. Doe, M.D.

3002 BROAD STREET ANYTOWN, ANYSTATE 00000

1 DATE 1/14/99 AGE 6

NAME Robert Stone

2 ADDRESS 605 Chatham Road
Trenton, N.J.

3 ℞

4 Poly-Vi-Flor
with Iron 0.5 mg.

5 Dispense #100 tabs

6 Sig. Chew 1 tab daily

Dr. Paula A. Doe Dr.

8 *Do Not Substitute* *Substitution Permissible*

7 Renew: 0 1 2 3 (4) 5 DEA #

FIGURE 1. A Sample Precompounded Prescription Order

2. **The Name, Address, and Age of the Patient** - This information serves to identify for whom the prescribed medication is intended. The full name of the patient may help to prevent a mixup of drugs within a household when, for example, a parent and child have the same name. If the patient's first name is not known or omitted, the use of the titles Mr., Mrs., Ms. or Miss is appropriate. Information regarding the patient's age should also be indicated, e.g., "adult," "child," or in the case of a young child, the exact age; this allows the pharmacist to monitor the prescribed dosage, especially since the pharmacokinetics of many drugs differ markedly in newborn, pediatric, adult, and geriatric patient populations.

3. **The Superscription** - This portion of the prescription refers to the symbol R_X, a contraction of the Latin verb *recipe*, meaning "take thou." It serves to introduce the drug(s) prescribed and the directions for use.

4. **The Inscription** - The name, strength and quantity of the desired drug is enclosed within this section of the prescription. Although drugs may be prescribed by any known name, i.e., chemical name, trivial name, nonproprietary name (more commonly referred to as the generic name) and manufacturer's proprietary (trade) name, most drugs are prescribed either by the trade name or by the generic name. Chemical and trivial names of drugs are generally not suitable for this purpose and are seldom used. When the trade name is written, the prescription must be filled with the product of the specified manufacturer, unless the prescriber and patient approved substitution with another brand. If the generic name is employed, the pharmacist can select from any of the available drug preparations. When two or more drugs are written on the same prescription for compounding purposes, the name and quantity of each should be listed on a separate line directly below the preceding one. To avoid confusion, the salt of a particular medicament should be clearly indicated if more than one is available, e.g., codeine <u>sulfate</u> or codeine <u>phosphate</u>. The quantities of the ingredients may be written in either the apothecary or metric system. The latter is more popular; it is used exclusively by official pharmaceutical reference texts, and in most cases, in medical schools, hospitals, and other health agencies.

The apothecary system is an older and less popular method of measurement; however, prescriptions are still written in this system and texts may, on occasion, report drug doses in apothecary units. For example, 1 fluid-ounce (apothecary) equals approximately 30 mL (metric) and 1 pint equals 473 mL.

Regardless of which system is employed on the prescription, most patients are more comfortable with household measures, especially with liquid medications. Although the sizes of the household teaspoon and tablespoon vary considerably, the standard household teaspoon should be regarded as containing 5 mL and the tablespoon, 15 mL. Standard disposable plastic teaspoons, tablespoons and graduated two fluid-ounce cups are available in an attempt to reduce liquid dose variability, and the use of these should be encouraged.

5. **The Subscription** - Directions to the pharmacist from the prescriber comprise this section of the prescription; these state the specific dosage form to be dispensed or the desired method of preparation. The subscription is usually a short phrase or sentence such as "Dispense 30 capsules" or "Dispense 90 mL" for a precompounded prescription or "Mix and prepare 10 suppositories" for an extemporaneous preparation.

6. **The Signa** - The directions to the patient are given in this part of the prescription and usually introduced by the latin *Signa* or *Sig.*, meaning "mark thou". These directions should be as clear and as complete as possible, so that the patient may easily follow the desired dosage schedule and receive the maximum benefit from the medication. Instructions should be provided as to the route of administration, the amount of drug to be taken, and the time and frequency of the dose. Phrases such as "take as directed" and "use as required" are not satisfactory instructions and should be avoided whenever possible.

Latin, often considered to be the language of the medical profession, was used extensively in writing prescription orders until the early part of the 20th century. Although prescription orders in the United States today are almost always written in English, many Latin words and phrases are retained and are commonly used (as abbreviations) in the Signa. Some of the more commonly-employed Latin terms and abbreviations are given in Table 1. Thus the Signa: "Caps 1 q.i.d. p.c. + H.S. c milk" translates to: "One capsule 4 times daily after meals and at bedtime with milk".

7. **The Renewal Information** - The wishes of the prescriber with regard to refilling the medication should be indicated on every prescription, and if renewals are authorized, the number of times should be designated. Prescription orders for drugs that bear the legend: "Caution: Federal law prohibits dispensing without prescription" may not be renewed without the expressed consent of the prescriber. Prescriptions for drugs covered under Schedule III or IV of the Controlled Substances Act of 1970 may be renewed, if so authorized, not more than five times within six months of date of issue; drugs within Schedule II may not be renewed.

8. **The Name of the Prescriber** - Although in most cases the prescriber's name and address are printed on the prescription blank, the signature of the prescriber affixed to the bottom completes and validates the prescription order. For prescriptions written on hospital prescription blanks, the prescriber must print (or stamp) his/her name on the document, as well as sign it. This is a safe-guard in case a question arises concerning any aspect of the prescription order, the printed name will make it easier to identify and contact the prescriber. On oral prescriptions, the pharmacist adds the prescriber's name to the prescription; however, Federal law requires that prescriptions for Schedule II drugs be validated by the full signature of the prescriber and his/her registered Drug Enforcement Administration (DEA) number. The prescriber's registered DEA number must appear on all prescriptions for drug covered under the Controlled Substances Act (see below).

CLASSES OF PRESCRIPTION ORDERS

Prescription orders may be divided into two general classes based on the availability of the medication. A **precompounded** prescription order requests a drug or a drug mixture prepared and supplied by a pharmaceutical company; prescriptions of this class require no pharmaceutical alteration by the pharmacist. The prescription order shown in Figure 1 is a precompounded prescription. An **extemporaneous** or **compounded** prescription order is one in which the drugs, doses and dosage form, as selected by the prescriber, must be prepared by the pharmacist. Figure 2 shows an example of an extemporaneous prescription order. Most prescriptions written today are of the precompounded type; however extemporaneous prescription orders are not uncommon, especially with liquid, cream, and ointment preparations.

CONTROLLED SUBSTANCES ACT

The legal aspects of prescription writing and dispensing are incorporated in various federal, state and local laws, which the medical practitioner must understand and observe; the strictest law regardless of governmental level, always takes precedence unless Federal Law is preemptive. In 1970, the Comprehensive Drug Abuse Prevention and Control Act, commonly called the Controlled Substances Act, was signed into law. This act imposes even more stringent controls on the distribution and use of all stimulant and depressant drugs and substances with the potential for abuse as designated by the Drug Enforcement Administration (DEA), U.S. Department of Justice. This act divides drugs with abuse potential into five categories or schedules as follows:

Schedule I (C-I) — Drugs in this schedule have a high potential for abuse and no currently accepted medical use in the United States. Examples of such drugs include heroin, marijuana, peyote, mescaline, some tetrahydrocannabinols, LSD, and various opioid derivatives. Substances listed in this

248

TABLE 1. COMMON LATIN ABBREVIATIONS

WORD OR PHRASE	ABBREVIATION	MEANING
Ad	Ad	Up to
Ana	aa	Of each
Ante cibos	a.c.	Before meals
Aqua	Aq.	Water
Aures utrae	a.u.	Each ear
Aurio dextra	a.d.	Right ear
Aurio laeva	a.l.	Left ear
Bis in die	b.i.d.	Twice a day
Capsula	Caps.	Capsule
Compositus	Comps.	Compounded
Cum	c	With
Et	Et	And
Gutta	Gtt.	A drop, drops
Hora somni	H.S.	At bedtime
Non repetatur	Non rep.	Do not repeat
Oculo utro	O.U.	Each eye
Oculus dexter	O.D.	Right eye
Oculus sinister	O.S.	Left eye
Per os	p.o.	By mouth
Post cibos	p.c.	After meals
Pro re nata	p.r.n.	When necessary
Quaque	q.	Each, every
Quantum satis	Q.S.	As much as is sufficient
Quarter in die	q.i.d.	Four times daily
Semis	ss	A half
Sine	s	Without
Statim	Stat.	Immediately
Tabella	tab	Tablet
Ter in die	t.i.d.	Three times daily
Ut dictum	Ut Dict.	As directed

TELEPHONE (215) 555-2474

John V. Smith, M.D.
Paula A. Doe, M.D.

3002 BROAD STREET   ANYTOWN, ANYSTATE 00000

DATE 1/14/99   AGE 3
NAME Sarah Lewis
ADDRESS 890 Main Street
Phila., Pa.

℞

Vioform cream 15 g
Hydrocortisone Cream 1%
Prep. 30 g Cream
Sig. Apply to affected
area B↓d

Dr. John Smith   Dr.
Do Not Substitute   Substitution
Permissible

Renew: 0 1 2 ③ 4 5   DEA #

FIGURE 2.   A Sample Extemporaneous Prescription Order

schedule are not for prescription use; they may be obtained for chemical analysis, research, or instruction purposes by submitting an application and a protocol of the proposed use to the DEA.

Schedule II (C-II) — The drugs in this schedule have a high abuse potential with severe psychological or physical dependence liability. Schedule II controlled substances consist of certain opioid drugs, preparations containing amphetamines or methamphetamines as the single active ingredient or in combination with each other, and certain sedatives. Examples of opioids included in this schedule are opium, morphine, codeine, hydromorphone (DILAUDID), methadone (DOLOPHINE), meperidine (DEMEROL), oxycodone (PERCODAN, PERCOCET), and oxymorphone (NUMORPHAN). Also included are stimulants, e.g., cocaine, dextroamphetamine (DEXEDRINE), methamphetamine (DESOXYN), methylphenidate (RITALIN), and depressants, e.g., amobarbital (AMYTAL SODIUM), pentobarbital (NEMBUTAL SODIUM), and secobarbital.

Schedule III (C-III) — The drugs in this schedule have a potential for abuse that is less than for those drugs in Schedules I and II. The use or abuse of these drugs may lead to low or moderate physical dependence or high psychological dependence. Included in this schedule, for example, are mazindol (SANOREX), and paregoric. Analgesic mixtures containing limited amounts of codeine phosphate (e.g., TYLENOL WITH CODEINE and EMPIRIN WITH CODEINE), or hydrocodone (e.g., ANEXSIA, BANCAP-HC, and LORTAB) or cough mixtures containing hydrocodone (e.g., HYCODAN and HYCOMINE) are contained within this schedule. Also included in this schedule are certain anabolic steroids (e.g., salts of nandrolone (DURABOLIN and DECA-DURABOLIN) and oxandrolone (OXANDRIN)).

Schedule IV (C-IV) — The drugs in this category have the potential for limited physical or psychological dependence and include phenobarbital, paraldehyde, chloral hydrate, ethchlorvynol (PLACIDYL), meprobamate (EQUANIL, MILTOWN), chlordiazepoxide (LIBRIUM), diazepam (VALIUM), clorazepate (TRANXENE), flurazepam (DALMANE), oxazepam (SERAX), clonazepam (KLONOPIN), lorazepam (ATIVAN), and salts of propoxyphene (DARVON and DARVON-N). Certain other mixtures are included; for example, the antidiarrheal MOTOFEN and the analgesic DARVOCET-N.

Schedule V (C-V) — Schedule V drugs have a potential for abuse that is less than those listed in Schedule IV. These consist of preparations containing moderate quantities of certain opioids for use in pain (i.e., buprenorphine (BUPRENEX)) or as antidiarrheals (e.g., diphenoxylate (LOMOTIL), or as antitussives (such as codeine-containing cough mixtures, e.g., ROBITUSSIN A-C) may be dispensed without a prescription order, provided that specified dispensing criteria are met by the pharmacist.

Every person involved in the manufacture, importing, exporting, distribution or dispensing of any Controlled Drug must obtain an annual registration from the DEA; therefore, a physician must be registered before he/she can administer or dispense any of the drugs listed in the abuse schedules. Furthermore, the physician's DEA registration number must be indicated on every prescription order for Controlled Substances.

Notes

INDEX

253

257

Dyphylline: 129

268

XYLOCAINE 2% VISCOUS: 71
Xylometazoline Hydrochloride: 108

ORDER FORM FOR HANDBOOKS

TITLE	PRICE × QUANTITY
Handbook of Commonly Prescribed Pediatric Drugs, Sixth Edition (1999), 272 pages ISBN 0-942447-27-1	$ 18.50 × _____ = $ _____._____
Handbook of Commonly Prescribed Drugs, Thirteenth Edition (1998), 294 pages ISBN 0-942447-25-5	$ 18.00 × _____ = $ _____._____
Drug Charts in Basic Pharmacology, Second Edition (1998), 304 pages ISBN 0-942447-26-3	$ 18.00 × _____ = $ _____._____
Antimicrobial Therapy in Primary Care Medicine (1997), 382 pages ISBN 0-942447-22-0	$ 16.50 × _____ = $ _____._____
Handbook of Common Orthopaedic Fractures, Third Edition (1997), 270 pages ISBN 0-942447-24-7	$ 17.00 × _____ = $ _____._____
Warning: Drugs in Sports (1995), 278 pages ISBN 0-942447-16-6	$ 14.50 × _____ = $ _____._____
Handbook of Commonly Prescribed Geriatric Drugs, First Edition (1993), 334 pages ISBN 0-942447-01-8	$ 15.00 × _____ = $ _____._____
	SUB-TOTAL = $ _____._____
Shipping and Handling Charge (see below)	= $ _____._____
PA Residents: Add 6% Sales Tax	= $ _____._____
	TOTAL = $ _____._____

Shipping and Handling Charges:

Add $ 5.50 for orders between $ 10.00 and $ 49.99
Add $ 8.00 for orders between $ 50.00 and $ 99.99
Add $10.00 for orders between $100.00 and $149.99
Add $12.00 for orders greater than $150.00

For mail orders for Handbooks, please complete the reverse side of this form.

ORDER FORM FOR TEXTBOOK
IN PHARMACOLOGY

TITLE	PRICE x QUANTITY
Basic Pharmacology in Medicine, Fourth Edition (1995), 880 pages ISBN 0-942447-04-2	$ 49.95 x _____ = $ _____.____
	SUB-TOTAL = $ _____.____
Shipping and Handling	= $ 5.50
PA Residents: Add 6% Sales Tax	= $ _____.____
	TOTAL = $ _____.____

Send mail orders for Handbooks or Textbook to:

MEDICAL SURVEILLANCE INC.
P.O. Box 480   Willow Grove, PA 19090

(PLEASE PRINT)

Name_____Degree_____

Organization_____

Street Address_____

City_____State_____Zip_____

Telephone Number_____

Payment: Check_____   VISA_____   MC_____   Discov_____   Am. Express_____

Credit Card No._____   Exp. Date_____

Signature_____

FOR FURTHER INFORMATION CALL: 800 - 417-3189 or 215 - 784-0976
FAX: 215 - 657-1475

ORDER FORM FOR HANDBOOKS

TITLE	PRICE x QUANTITY
Handbook of Commonly Prescribed Pediatric Drugs, Sixth Edition (1999), 272 pages ISBN 0-942447-27-1	$ 18.50 x _____ = $ _____._____
Handbook of Commonly Prescribed Drugs, Thirteenth Edition (1998), 294 pages ISBN 0-942447-25-5	$ 18.00 x _____ = $ _____._____
Drug Charts in Basic Pharmacology, Second Edition (1998), 304 pages ISBN 0-942447-26-3	$ 18.00 x _____ = $ _____._____
Antimicrobial Therapy in Primary Care Medicine (1997), 382 pages ISBN 0-942447-22-0	$ 16.50 x _____ = $ _____._____
Handbook of Common Orthopaedic Fractures, Third Edition (1997), 270 pages ISBN 0-942447-24-7	$ 17.00 x _____ = $ _____._____
Warning: Drugs in Sports (1995), 278 pages ISBN 0-942447-16-6	$ 14.50 x _____ = $ _____._____
Handbook of Commonly Prescribed Geriatric Drugs, First Edition (1993), 334 pages ISBN 0-942447-01-8	$ 15.00 x _____ = $ _____._____
	SUB-TOTAL = $ _____._____
Shipping and Handling Charge (see below)	= $ _____._____
PA Residents: Add 6% Sales Tax	= $ _____._____
	TOTAL = $ _____._____

Shipping and Handling Charges:

Add $ 5.50 for orders between $ 10.00 and $ 49.99
Add $ 8.00 for orders between $ 50.00 and $ 99.99
Add $10.00 for orders between $100.00 and $149.99
Add $12.00 for orders greater than $150.00

For mail orders for Handbooks, please complete the reverse side of this form.

ORDER FORM FOR TEXTBOOK
IN PHARMACOLOGY

TITLE	PRICE x QUANTITY		
Basic Pharmacology in Medicine, Fourth Edition (1995), 880 pages ISBN 0-942447-04-2	$ 49.95 x _____ = $ _____._____		
	SUB-TOTAL	=	$ _____._____
Shipping and Handling		=	$ __5.50__
PA Residents: Add 6% Sales Tax		=	$ _____._____
	TOTAL	=	$ _____._____

Send mail orders for Handbooks or Textbook to:

MEDICAL SURVEILLANCE INC.
P.O. Box 480   Willow Grove, PA 19090

(PLEASE PRINT)

Name_____Degree_____

Organization_____

Street Address_____

City_____State_____Zip_____

Telephone Number_____

Payment: Check_____ VISA_____ MC_____ Discov_____ Am. Express_____

Credit Card No._____ Exp. Date_____

Signature_____

FOR FURTHER INFORMATION CALL: 800 - 417-3189 or 215 - 784-0976
FAX: 215 - 657-1475

ORDER FORM FOR HANDBOOKS

TITLE	PRICE x QUANTITY
Handbook of Commonly Prescribed Pediatric Drugs, Sixth Edition (1999), 272 pages ISBN 0-942447-27-1	$ 18.50 x ____ = $ ____.____
Handbook of Commonly Prescribed Drugs, Thirteenth Edition (1998), 294 pages ISBN 0-942447-25-5	$ 18.00 x ____ = $ ____.____
Drug Charts in Basic Pharmacology, Second Edition (1998), 304 pages ISBN 0-942447-26-3	$ 18.00 x ____ = $ ____.____
Antimicrobial Therapy in Primary Care Medicine (1997), 382 pages ISBN 0-942447-22-0	$ 16.50 x ____ = $ ____.____
Handbook of Common Orthopaedic Fractures, Third Edition (1997), 270 pages ISBN 0-942447-24-7	$ 17.00 x ____ = $ ____.____
Warning: Drugs in Sports (1995), 278 pages ISBN 0-942447-16-6	$ 14.50 x ____ = $ ____.____
Handbook of Commonly Prescribed Geriatric Drugs, First Edition (1993), 334 pages ISBN 0-942447-01-8	$ 15.00 x ____ = $ ____.____
	SUB-TOTAL = $ ____.____
Shipping and Handling Charge (see below)	= $ ____.____
PA Residents: Add 6% Sales Tax	= $ ____.____
	TOTAL = $ ____.____

Shipping and Handling Charges:

Add $ 5.50 for orders between $ 10.00 and $ 49.99
Add $ 8.00 for orders between $ 50.00 and $ 99.99
Add $10.00 for orders between $100.00 and $149.99
Add $12.00 for orders greater than $150.00

For mail orders for Handbooks, please complete the reverse side of this form.

ORDER FORM FOR TEXTBOOK
IN PHARMACOLOGY

TITLE	PRICE x QUANTITY
Basic Pharmacology in Medicine, Fourth Edition (1995), 880 pages ISBN 0-942447-04-2	$ 49.95 x _____ = $ _____.____
	SUB-TOTAL = $ _____.____
Shipping and Handling	= $ 5.50
PA Residents: Add 6% Sales Tax	= $ _____.____
	TOTAL = $ _____.____

Send mail orders for Handbooks or Textbook to:

MEDICAL SURVEILLANCE INC.
P.O. Box 480   Willow Grove, PA 19090

(PLEASE PRINT)

Name_____Degree_____

Organization_____

Street Address_____

City_____State_____Zip_____

Telephone Number_____

Payment: Check____   VISA____   MC____   Discov____   Am. Express____

Credit Card No._____   Exp. Date_____

Signature_____

FOR FURTHER INFORMATION CALL: 800 - 417-3189 or 215 - 784-0976
FAX: 215 - 657-1475

REQUEST FOR INFORMATION

If you wish to be placed on a mailing list for information concerning new publications and updates, please fill out the form below and mail to:

MEDICAL SURVEILLANCE INC.
P.O. Box 480   Willow Grove, PA 19090

(PLEASE PRINT)

Name_____

Organization_____

Street Address_____

City_____State_____

Zip Code_____

Telephone Number (Optional)_____

FOR FURTHER INFORMATION CALL:
800 - 417-3189 or 215 - 784-0976

E-Mail us at msi@juno.com

Visit Us on the **World Wide Web** at
hhtp://www.medicalsurveillance.com

REQUEST FOR INFORMATION

If you wish to be placed on a mailing list for information concerning new publications and updates, please fill out the form below and mail to:

MEDICAL SURVEILLANCE INC.
P.O. Box 480   Willow Grove, PA 19090

(PLEASE PRINT)

Name_____

Organization_____

Street Address_____

City_____State_____

Zip Code_____

Telephone Number (Optional)_____

FOR FURTHER INFORMATION CALL:
800 - 417-3189 or 215 - 784-0976

E-Mail us at msi@juno.com

Visit Us on the **World Wide Web** at
hhtp://www.medicalsurveillance.com